CARE
AND FEEDING
OF THE
BRAIN

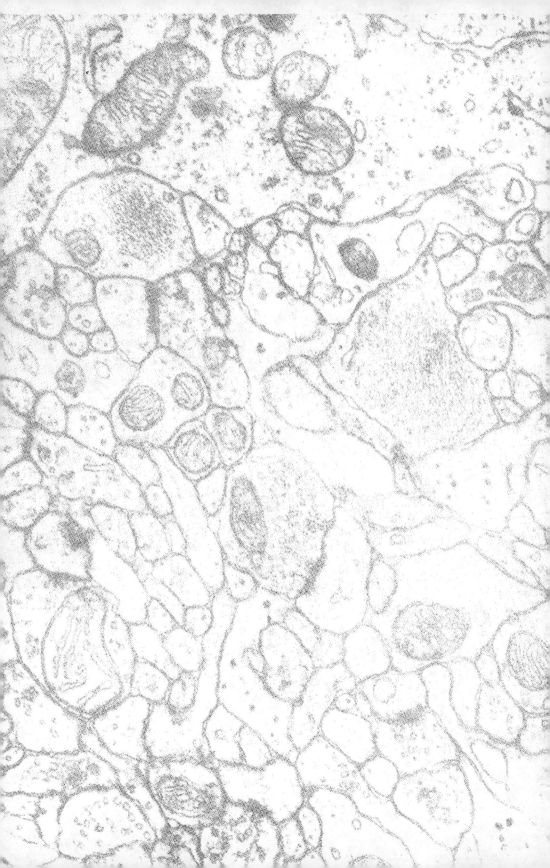

CARE AND FEEDING OF THE BRAIN

A GUIDE TO YOUR GRAY MATTER

JACK MAGUIRE
and THE PHILIP LEIF GROUP, INC.

DOUBLEDAY
NEW YORK   LONDON   TORONTO   SYDNEY   AUCKLAND

PUBLISHED BY DOUBLEDAY
a division of Bantam Doubleday Dell Publishing Group, Inc.
666 Fifth Avenue, New York, New York 10103

DOUBLEDAY and the portrayal of an anchor
with a dolphin are trademarks of Doubleday,
a division of Bantam Doubleday Dell
Publishing Group, Inc.

Library of Congress Cataloging-in-Publication Data

Maguire, Jack.
  Care and feeding of the brain : a guide to your gray matter / by
Jack Maguire.—
      p.   cm.
  1. Brain—Popular works.   I. Title.
QP376.M286   1990
612.8'2—dc20   89-27385
                                                               CIP

ISBN 0-385-26411-9
ISBN 978-0-385-26412-9

Art Director: Carol Malcolm

Book Design by Julie McIntyre

Illustrations by Jackie Aher

147146388

This book is dedicated
to my good friends
Philip Lief and Susan Osborn

Among the many individuals
who helped me to put this book together
I am especially grateful
to Jamie Rothstein
and to my editor, Kara Leverte.
Their patience, skill and
creativity were invaluable.

CONTENTS

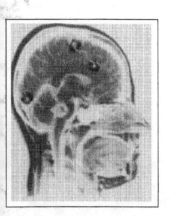

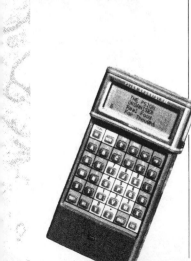

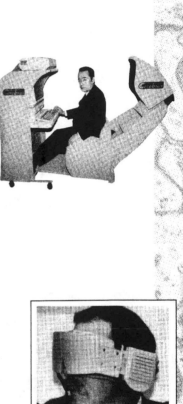

CARE
AND FEEDING
OF THE
BRAIN

1
HOW THE BRAIN WORKS

hen we're worried about cellulite, love handles, a weak grip, a thickening midriff, or a sagging pec deck, we know what to do—go to a gym. But what do we do if we're worried about worry itself, or about insomnia, emotional exhaustion, a faulty memory, a sluggish imagination, a shaky attention span?

Once there didn't seem to be much we could do for these kinds of brain-related problems. Reluctant to run away to the Fiji Islands or commit ourselves to years of expensive therapy, we would decide to ignore problems that didn't show up in the mirror: out of sight, out of, well, mind. Now that's no longer the situation. For the sake of a fine-tuned brain, we can do the same thing we do for a fine-tuned body: go to a gym.

"Brain spas," as they're called, are sprouting up across the United States. Like physical fitness centers, they offer state-of-the-art machinery to help patrons get back into shape. There is, however, a critical and delightful difference. You don't have to sweat and strain to work on mind machines. Instead, they work on you, employing various combinations of light, sound, and motion (or, alternatively, sensory deprivation) to lower stress, induce calm, break through memory blocks, sharpen the intellect, and stimulate creativity. While science has yet to grant them an unqualified endorsement, they are legitimate heirs of the same technological revolution that brought us the biofeedback devices of the 1960s and the computerized diagnostic and treatment equipment of the 1970s and 1980s—all standard gear in today's hospitals and neurological laboratories.

Fueling this astounding revolution in technology has been an even greater revolution in knowledge. We've learned more about the brain in the past thirty years than in the rest of human history; and the result has been an explosive growth in our understanding of how to use food, drugs, education, training, and even machinery to

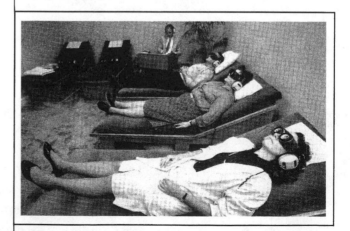

"Building a burn" at a brain spa in San Fransisco is no sweat at all. Here clients are hooked to a Synchro-Energizer (see page 65).

make the most of our brain's potential. *Care and Feeding of the Brain* is designed to introduce you to this exciting new frontier of brain science and technology and to help you capitalize on its discoveries.

In contrast to the wonder it arouses, the physical brain itself looks comically insignificant. About three pounds in weight and the size of two fists, it resembles an upscaled, jellied walnut. But that jellied walnut has been 500 million years in the making, and it's by far the most remarkable organ in our body, both architecturally and functionally. More than anything else, giving it the attention it deserves requires appreciating why it is so extraordinary.

First, let's consider the brain's intricate assortment of parts:

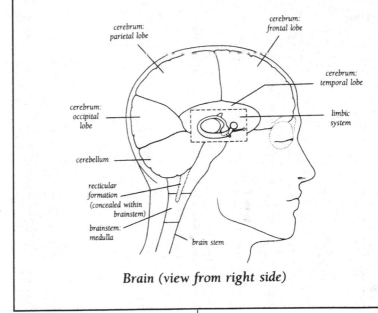

Brain (view from right side)

Brain Stem. Located at the top of our spine (just below our ears), the brain stem is the oldest part of our brain. In evolutionary terms, it is virtually identical to the brain of a reptile; hence, scientists refer to it as the "reptilian" brain. It houses the reticular formation, which alerts the brain to incoming data from the body and governs basic activities like consciousness, breathing, and heart rate.

Cerebellum. Directly behind the brain stem lies the cerebellum. It's primarily concerned with our body's movement through space, helping us to assume postures and maintain muscle coordination. It also contains a memory bank for simple learned motor responses, such as pulling our finger away from a flame.

The Limbic System. The limbic system is an interconnected group of structures perched on top of the brain stem. Because it contains the mechanisms that make an organism warm-blooded, it's known as the "mammalian" brain. In addition to controlling body temperature, blood pressure, and blood sugar, it's the processor of many of our emotional reactions, especially life-sustaining ones having to do with sex and aggression (the so-called "fight-or-flight" response).

Cerebrum. When we look at a brain in a jar of formaldehyde, we mainly see the cerebrum, and so we think of this structure as "the brain." It's split into left and right hemispheres (the halves of the "walnut") joined by a bridge of nerve fibers, the corpus callosum. Covering these two hemispheres is a one-eighth-inch-thick layer of rumpled gray matter called the cortex.

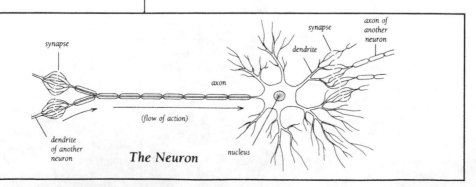

synapse

dendrite of another neuron

axon

(flow of action)

nucleus

synapse

dendrite

axon of another neuron

The Neuron

The cortex makes us human beings. It can be divided into four areas or lobes: (1) frontal, having to do with decision-making, problem-solving, and will; (2) parietal, having to do with the reception of sensory information; (3) occipital, having to do with vision; and (4) temporal, having to do with hearing, memory, and language.

✦✦✦✦✦✦✦✦✦

Now let's consider the fascinating way the brain does its work. The main operational unit is the microscopic nerve cell, or neuron, of which there are an estimated 100 billion in the average brain, all linked together in a highly sensitive network. When one neuron is stimulated by another, here's what happens: An electrical impulse travels through the branchlike dendrites and down the long, trunklike axon to the nucleus; the impulse directs the nucleus to release appropriate chemicals, called neurotransmitters or neurochemicals; these neurotransmitters flow into the gap, called the synapse, between one neuron and a neighboring neuron, where they activate receptors on the neighboring neuron's dendrites.

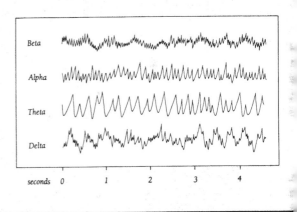

The brain's overall electrical activity can be mechanically recorded as a brain-wave pattern. Different brain-wave patterns reflect different states of consciousness. Relatively rapid Beta waves are associated with normal arousal. Slower Alpha waves indicate a relaxed, meditative state. Theta waves, which are slower yet, represent drowsiness or deep reverie. Delta waves, the slowest waves of all, represent sleep.

Thus, in a unique and still mysterious electrochemical process, one neuron communicates with another and vast systems of neurons process individual brain activities. Some extremely elementary functions are localized in certain sections of the brain; but most functions necessary for conducting intelligent life involve different parts of the brain cooperating. When your brain registers the image of a stop sign, for example, only a certain, site-specific segment of the neural network might be activated. But translating that stop sign into its meaning—"stop"—and then going through the mental and physical tasks required to respond to that meaning may shake up the brain's neural network from one end to the other.

There's some degree of structural regularity from brain to brain, but individual brains are as different as individual faces or fingerprints, from the size, weight, and proportion of brain parts to the groove pattern on the cerebrum. The precise way the brain functions also varies from individual to individual, according to genetic inheritance, life experiences, diet, drug exposure, and even the quality of air intake. Each of us truly has his or her own genius, as well as a unique responsibility for protecting and cultivating that genius.

Brief as this overview of the brain may be, it gives you some idea of the complexities involved in how the brain works. Succeeding chapters of *Care and Feeding of the Brain* will help you understand, facilitate, and enhance specific functional aspects of the brain's labor—namely, consciousness, memory, intelligence, emotions, and the mind-body connection. In this chapter, you'll learn more about brain operations as a whole. Separate discussions will help you make sense of the differences between right vs. left brains, male vs. female brains, and sane vs. insane brains. They'll tell you the causes and cures of headaches and common addictions. They'll give you more insight into how your genes and your environment meet to engineer your particular brain power and personality. And they'll introduce you to some major artillery in the new arsenal of brain machines.

What's the Real Difference Between My Right Brain and My Left Brain?

Nothing is so strong as an idea whose time has come, and nothing proves this more than the heavy impact of the

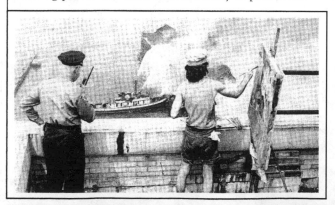

An accident at a pier: The cop on the left regards it as a problem-solving crisis. The artist on the right sees it as an artistic challenge. Such is the stereotypical view of right brain versus left brain perspectives.

"left brain versus right brain" concept on popular culture over the past twenty years. As the allegedly well-informed man or woman on the street would have it, the left hemisphere of the cerebrum is logical, the right hemisphere is intuitive, and people need to utilize both hemispheres to have a world-class, "whole-brain" intelligence. Fortune 500 corporations proudly sponsor training programs to unite "right-brain" creativity with "left-brain" business savvy. Hip advertisers borrow the idea to sell beef ("the left brain knows it's good for you, the right brain just knows it tastes good"). Progressive schools make sure they supplement their students' "left-brain" learning activities like reading with "right-brain" learning activities like drawing.

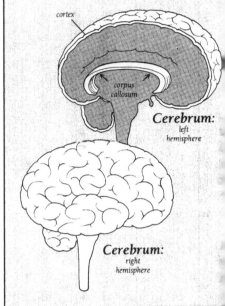

cortex

corpus callosum

Cerebrum:
left
hemisphere

Cerebrum:
right
hemisphere

Although these corporations, advertisers, and students often reap tangible benefits in the name of the left brain versus right brain idea, the truth that lies behind that idea is not nearly as black and white as they paint it. True, the cortex of the cerebrum's left hemisphere does tend to assume major responsibility for the so-called analytical functions: understanding language, speaking, computing, and judging time and sequence. True, the cortex of the cerebrum's right hemisphere does tend to assume major responsibility for the so-called imaginative functions: recognizing faces, reconstructing melodies, visualizing images. But the two hemispheres are far more similar than they are different, and virtually every mental process requires that they work in concert. The notion of a mute but magically sensitive right brain forever shouted down by a clever but cold-hearted left brain is irresistibly romantic—especially to a generation of weary technocrats—but it's also irrefutably false.

Charting the functional areas of the brain has been a scientific preoccupation and a popular craze for two centuries, since the French surgeon La Peyronie first cataloged the strange behaviors that follow specific brain injuries. In 1819, Dr. Franz Joseph Gall invented the science of phrenology, whereby the brain is divided into twenty-seven separate "faculty areas," and an individual's personality is supposedly read by feeling the corresponding bumps on his or her skull. Phrenology was definitely an idea whose time had come: It took fifty years for well-educated people to stop judging character by forehead bulges. By then, brain science was astir with the more conclusive findings of Dr. Paul Broca, a neuroanatomist who isolated an area on the left hemisphere that can be demonstrably associated with the ability to speak.

Finally, during the 1960s, Dr. Roger W. Sperry published his breakthrough research on the functional differences between the brain's right hemisphere and left hemisphere. Sperry was able to establish these differences by studying the brains of epileptics whose hemispheres had been surgically disconnected to prevent seizures. Since the left hemisphere of the brain controls the right side of the body and vice versa, a great many of Sperry's experiments featured playing the right side of the body against the left. In one series of exercises, for instance, he simultaneously flashed an image of a square to the subject's right brain only (via the left eye) and an image of a circle to the subject's left brain only (via the right eye). When the subject was asked to state what he or she saw (a left-brain activity), the subject would say, "A circle." However, when the subject was asked to draw a picture of what he or she saw (a right-brain activity), the subject would draw a square.

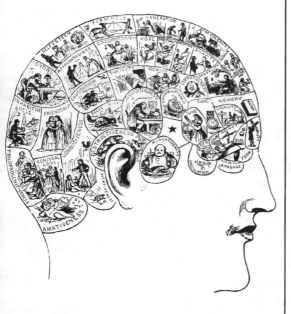

This 1869 phrenological chart purports to show the locations of different mental functions within the brain.

In cases of completely severed hemispheres, like the one just mentioned, left brain versus right brain differences are much more apparent—at least in the laboratory; in daily life, two severed hemispheres will cooperate in performing almost all normal tasks, despite the lack of a connective bridge of nerve fibers. Certain nonepileptic individuals whose hemispheres are *not* disconnected can still suffer minor glitches in hemisphere interaction that also bring out right-brain, left-brain differences: Dyslexia and stuttering are two of the more prevalent malfunctions of this type.

Right-brain versus left-brain operation varies slightly according to whether a person is right-handed or left-handed. No one knows why one person in ten is fully left-handed, but we do know that about 60 percent of "lefties," like "righties," process speech in the left hemisphere, while the other 40 percent use both sides of the brain. This is one indication that each of the brain's hemispheres has the potential of processing *any* function. The brain frequently takes advantage of this potential when a particular brain area is injured by an external blow or a stroke, or when biology throws the brain a curve. It's even possible that the cerebrum evolved into two almost identical parts just so there would be a "spare brain" in case of accidents.

The latest scientific testing indicates that the two hemispheres may be specialized not only for thinking but also for emoting. In 1987, Yale researchers Geoffrey Ahern and Gary Schwartz attached thirty-three subjects to machines that measured electrical activity in various parts of the brain. Then they asked each subject sixty questions carefully designed to evoke different moods. They found that the frontal lobes of the left hemisphere displayed more electrical activity when the subjects experienced positive emotions (like happiness or enthusiasm) and the frontal lobes of the right hemisphere displayed more electrical activity when the subjects experienced negative emotions (like sadness or disgust). As you might expect, scientists in general experience mixed emotions when they are queried about the significance of this research.

Meanwhile, the myth that the left brain is a calculator and that the right brain is a crystal ball continues to hold sway. And the myth is popular precisely because it does people good: It gets them to experiment with contrasting ways of using their "brains." As children, most of us went through a period of trying to train ourselves to be ambidextrous (able to write or perform other manipulating activities with both hands), and yet we dropped the effort after a while because it seemed silly. Now we can choose among a wide range of intriguing and socially encouraged options for developing better right and left brain coordination. Dr. Win Wenger, a Maryland educator, calls this endeavor "pole-bridging," and offers as an example learning to sight-read music (a left-brain activity) at the same time as learning to sing (a right-brain activity). It may not accomplish anything from a scientific perspective, but it stands a good chance of making some beautiful music.

MALE VS. FEMALE BRAINS

}FACT
}OR
}FOLK-
}LORE?

Everyone agrees that males and females are different—the difference
speaks for itself in the intensely dramatic
war and peace between the sexes. Few issues are more
divisive, however, than the debate about whether a male
brain differs from a female brain. True, a man's brain
tends to be bigger than a woman's brain simply because
men tend to be bigger than women; but as far as brain
power is concerned, does size have any bearing on performance? And if size doesn't, is there any other gender-
specific factor that does?

Given the way the brain operates—not through a bulk
accumulation of facts and strengths but through electrochemical processing—the size differential between a
man's brain and a woman's brain is meaningless. Nevertheless, brain researchers in the 1970s and 1980s have
managed to identify some distinctions that are significant.

**The cortex of the left hemisphere tends to be thicker
(or more "mature") in a female brain; the cortex of the
right hemisphere tends to be thicker in a male brain.**
As a result, women are predisposed to be better with
words than men. On the average they speak earlier, learn
languages more easily, and are more successful at rapidly
repeating tongue twisters like "a box of mixed biscuits in
a biscuit mixer" than their male peers. They also excel in
fine motor control, which translates into better penman-
ship—or, rather, pen*person*ship—among other things.
Men, by contrast, are inclined to be better than women in
spatial functions, such as visualizing a floorplan or negoti-
ating a maze, and in tasks involving control of the large
muscles, such as beating a drum or hitting a target with
darts.

The corpus callosum—the network of fibers connecting the left hemisphere with the right hemisphere—is proportionately larger in a female brain than it is in a male brain. For centuries, doctors have observed that women recover more quickly than men from most forms of brain damage, but it wasn't until recently that they figured out why: Women's right and left hemispheres are more closely interconnected, so one hemisphere can more easily compensate for damage to the other.

Up until puberty, the right and left hemispheres in all human beings become increasingly specialized, each one taking more and more responsibility for certain functions. As this happens, the corpus callosum gets thinner and thinner. Since women as a rule reach puberty earlier than men, their brains have less time to specialize. Men, with their more specialized hemispheres, not only undergo more difficulty recovering from brain damage compared to women, but they're also far more frequently the victims of dyslexia, stuttering, delayed reactions, autism, and hyperactivity.

Dr. Jerre Levy of the University of Chicago theorizes that the stronger corpus callosum link in the female brain could explain "women's intuition," as well as men's apparent superiority in mechanics and math. A woman, she suggests, might be better able to integrate all the details and nuances of a particular situation, due to the fact that her two hemispheres can communicate with each other more rapidly. The more "compartmentalized" male brain might be better able to focus with precision on a limited number of relevant details.

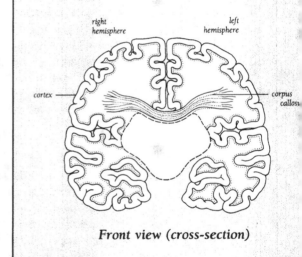

Front view (cross-section)

Brain tissue is "masculinized" or "feminized" by sex hormones. Why do only male birds sing? Dr. Fernando Nottebohm of New York City's Rockefeller University discovered that the male sex hormone testosterone stimulates the growth of a brain-cell cluster in the forebrain of the male songbird that doesn't exist in the forebrain of the female songbird (paradoxically, a nonsinging songbird).

This brain-cell cluster gives the male the smarts and the muscle control to make music, which it needs to do to attract a mate.

In human beings, scientists contend, sex hormones also stamp a brain "male" or "female." Dr. Doreen Kimura, a psychologist at the University of Western Ontario, recently studied 200 women and found that they performed better on tasks involving verbal skill or muscle coordination when their estrogen levels were high (just before ovulation) than when their levels were low (at the beginning of the menstrual cycle and shortly before menstruation itself). Alternatively, they did better on tasks involving spatial relationships when their estrogen levels were low than when their levels were high. Putting these results together with other research findings, scientists are now deciding that sex-specific hormones help carve out the brain's transmission system and, therefore, facilitate its operation. Consequently, males and females do process an indeterminate amount of functions differently. One human sex may well "sing songs" that the other human sex doesn't. If so, we don't yet know the specific melodies.

◆◆◆◆◆◆◆◆◆◆

These latest discoveries that the male brain and the female brain are, once and for all, different haven't ended the grand debate; they've only changed it. Marilyn Fitterman of the National Organization for Women worries that the data "could fall into the category of 'why a woman can't be president.'" Scientists warn against this kind of crude misinterpretation, emphasizing that only part of the difference between males and females in any one skill area is due to the anatomical and chemical makeup of their brains. The other part—as much as 80 percent by many estimates—depends on the individual's level of expectation, the degree to which he or she is encouraged, and the style and extent of his or her education. Many men, for example, are terrible at map-reading (a spatial task); many women read maps effortlessly.

More to the point, potential brain-influenced skill discrepancies between one sex in general and the other sex in general are just not that great. Dr. Roger Gorski of the University of California at Los Angeles sums it up best:

"There are subtle differences in the brain functions of individuals. That doesn't mean that a woman can't solve the
subtle problems of being president." It also doesn't mean
that a man can't bungle them!

How Much of My Brain Power and Personality Is Inherited?

James Lewis and James Springer are identical twins who
were separated shortly after birth and never knew about
each other's existence. When they were reunited at the
age of forty in 1979, they were dumbfounded at the simi-
larities in their lives. Both twins had married and di-
vorced women named Linda and were then in their
second marriages to women named Betty. Each had
undergone police training. They enjoyed the same hobbies
(woodworking and golf), drove the same model blue
Chevrolet, vacationed at the same beach outside St.
Petersburg, Florida, and owned dogs named Toy.

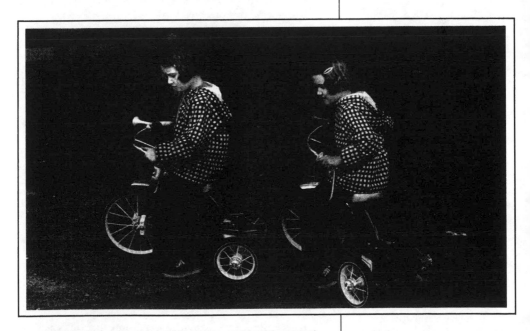

Identical twins tend to assume similar postures and facial expressions to accompany the same experience, even if the twins are raised separately and never meet each other.

While it's impossible to explain many of the correspondencies in their lives, it's also impossible to dismiss them all as coincidences. Obviously some factor tied to their biological status as twins led them to experience similar fates.

In the study of inherited traits and tendencies, two heads are dramatically better than one, especially if those two heads belong to twins separated at birth and raised in different environments. The fact that identical twins share the exact same genes helps researchers observing them to make more authoritative distinctions between the apparent products of nature and the apparent products of nurture. If the identical twins under observation were reared separately, these kinds of distinctions stand out all the more clearly. According to Dr. Thomas J. Bouchard, Jr., director of the Minnesota Center for Twin and Adoption Research at the University of Minnesota, the life histories of such twins reveal "things you would never think of looking at if you were going to study the genetics of behavior."

Through his meticulous, firsthand analysis of the lifestyles and psychological profiles of 350 pairs of identical twins reared apart, Bouchard came to the following conclusions regarding how much of our brain power and personality is inherited.

Man's mind,
stretched to a new idea, never goes back to
its original dimension.
—Oliver Wendell Holmes

• Most of an individual's leadership ability is inherited: based on tests, roughly 60 percent.
• In terms of an individual's capacity for aggression, orderliness, social closeness, and intellectual achievement, upbringing is more important than biology (tests suggested only a 33 to 48 percent genetic contribution).
• Shyness is one of the traits most strongly linked to heredity. It appears to be the effect of a brain-driven physiological system that is extremely sensitive and, therefore, compels the individual to be more cautious and subdued.
• Fears and phobias are also highly subject to being inherited, although the mechanisms that put this inheritance into action are obscure.

To dispel any inherited or noninherited fears we may have that our lives are programmed from birth, Bouchard and other experts on the subject assure us that the way genes work to shape our destiny is very indirect. An individual's genes do not dictate real-life brain power and personality; they merely influence what kinds of environments (i.e., work, play, living, and social setups) an individual will seek, which will, in turn, determine his or her ongoing brain power applications and personality manifestations. By the same token, genes are only one factor among many that will mold an individual's brain power and personality in environments that are not necessarily of his or her choosing.

In other words, neither biology nor sociology has the final say in what we do with our brains and our personalities. A born leader may never get much scope for leading if he or she is compelled through circumstances to remain impoverished, isolated, or dominated by an even stronger leader. A born poet may unknowingly channel that creative energy into running a business, so that he or she can realize an even stronger proclivity for social success. If that latent poet is subsequently disabled and housebound, then the poetic urge may take over.

Focusing on the unusual number of correspondencies between the Springer–Lewis twins, we can speculate that their mutual interest in woodworking and golf probably sprang from bred-in-the-bone likenesses that were physical as well as psychological: They were both encouraged by nature to choose activities that not only were solitary and easygoing, but also gave them something to do with their hands. Likewise, they may have been enticed by their genes to marry at an early age, before they were emotionally mature enough to make a marriage work. This would account for the fact that both of them went through a divorce. What remains truly weird is the Linda–Linda, Betty–Betty, Toy–Toy name connection, unless you hypothesize (as Bouchard does not) that the twins were born with ears attuned to those specific sounds!

We are what we think.
All that we are arises with our thoughts.
With our thoughts we create the world.
—Gautama Buddha

ADDICTION

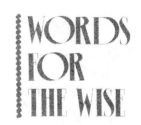

WORDS FOR THE WISE

When Kitty Dukakis, wife of Massachusetts Governor Michael Dukakis, publicly confessed her addiction to alcohol three months after her husband's unsuccessful 1988 run for the presidency, friends and strangers alike were shocked. How could an addict maintain such a productive work schedule? After kicking a twenty-six-year amphetamine habit seven years previously, how could Dukakis allow herself to develop yet another addiction?

Even scientists who specialize in substance abuse have a hard time defining addiction, let alone how addiction and addicts operate. We talk fast and loose about addiction to food, sex, gambling, or shopping; but, from a scientific perspective, these latter "addictions" are due to compulsive behaviors, with no discernible roots in brain functioning. An out-of-control reliance on alcohol or any other drug is another matter. Here science is able to draw the line: Medically speaking, addiction is a chemical dependence. The brain comes to need the offending drug more and more in order to avoid escalating physical pain.

Different chemical compounds affect the brain in different ways to cause addiction. Here is some information on the most common addictive substances.

Caffeine. The caffeine in coffee works on the brain stem's reticular formation, which controls consciousness. It enlivens the flow of electrochemical connections among brain cells, making the drinker more alert. Consistent intake of caffeine (a cup or more of coffee a day) can gear the brain to await the caffeine stimulus before it responds with wakefulness. Sudden withdrawal from long-term caffeine intake can cause headaches and dizziness.

Nicotine. The nicotine in cigarettes causes a general, as yet undefined alteration in brain chemicals that somehow produces a feeling of well-being. Most likely, a smoker continues to smoke to achieve the same brain chemical activity he or she has come to associate with the pleasing ritual of smoking. Scientists still question whether nicotine is truly addictive, since the level of dependence hinges so strongly on psychological factors; but withdrawal does cause physical pains. In May 1988, U.S. Surgeon General C. Everett Koop published what he termed "overwhelming evidence that tobacco is addicting in the same sense as drugs such as heroin and cocaine."

Alcohol. Alcohol works on the brain stem's reticular formation to create a "depressed" or less alert form of consciousness. The immediate effect is a "high" due to a release of tension. This is followed by relaxation and a loss of inhibitions. It's unclear precisely what constitutes alcohol addiction; but the bottom line is that the abusive drinker's brain grows so used to a certain level of alcohol that being without it becomes unbearable.

Evidence is now emerging that some individuals are genetically predisposed to alcoholism. The inherited trait seems to be a decreased reaction to drinking during the first three to five drinks; because the drinker's brain is slow to indicate drunkenness, the drinker consumes more alcohol than he or she should. People of Mongoloid descent (Asiatics and Native Americans) are genetically inclined to experience drunkenness earlier and more powerfully than drinkers of the other races, which may or may not put them at higher risk for alcoholism.

Heroin and Morphine. In the 1970s, scientists discovered that opiates like heroin and morphine work because brain cells contain built-in "opiate receptors," passages through which only opiate compounds can gain entry and perform their pain-killing, euphoria-spreading magic. Why should the brain have such a system, researchers wondered, unless the brain manufactures its own opiates? Sure enough, the brain does produce its own opiates: endorphins.

When we go into a merciful state of shock, it's because endorphins have sent us there. When we thrill and chill to our favorite music, we're responding to a sudden rush of endorphins. When mothers give birth, their endorphin level rises ten times above normal, for their own benefit as well as their child's. Endorphins may even be released by the stress of exercise, accounting for feelings like "runner's high."

Introducing outside opiates to this system wreaks havoc. The body requires increasingly higher doses to achieve the same degree of pleasure; and if the same degree of pleasure isn't obtained, the resulting pain gets progressively greater. Withdrawal can cause extreme physical suffering, hallucinations, and even death.

Cocaine. As in schizophrenia and Parkinson's disease, the key neurochemical involved in cocaine addiction is dopamine (see "Schizophrenics," page 26). Cocaine slows down the transmission of dopamine from one brain cell to another. Thus dopamine spends a longer time stimulating each brain cell receptor, and the effect, for some reason, is pleasurable. Sooner or later, dopamine receptors get desensitized through this process, and it requires a heavier dose of cocaine to create the same sensation. Big highs are followed by ever bigger lows. Withdrawal can be just as harsh as it is for opiates.

Amphetamines and Barbiturates. Amphetamines ("uppers" or "pep pills") act like the neurochemical adrenaline: They stimulate brain activities across the board. Unfortunately, amphetamines cannot be naturally reabsorbed when they're no longer needed. The crash from up to down is severe, and so an addictive use pattern sets in to keep the buzz going. Long-term use can cause convulsions, delusions, and psychoses. So can withdrawal. Barbiturates ("downers" or "tranquilizers") mimic brain chemicals that cause sedation. The general pattern of addiction and withdrawal is the same as it is for amphetamines.

Marijuana. The active chemical in marijuana—commonly abbreviated as THC—overstimulates sensory nerves in the brain stem, which explains why users become more acutely sensitive to what they touch, taste, see, hear, and smell, and why they occasionally hallucinate. The medical community is sharply divided over whether marijuana is *chemically* addictive, although most experts agree that it is *psychologically* addictive. Prolonged consumption leads to diminished short-term memory, loss of initiative, and, possibly, a weakening of the immune system. Withdrawal is characterized by irritability, dietary cravings, and/or headaches.

◆◆◆◆◆◆◆◆◆◆◆

A behavioral profile of a typical addict or addiction-prone person is impossible to draw. Some turn on to escape depression. Some turn on sheerly for the high. Some don't even know they're turning on; instead, the drugs they're taking silently turn on them. "Anyone with a healthy, functioning nervous system is vulnerable," says Jack Henningfield of the National Institute on Drug Abuse. "What we see is an interaction of personality, environment, biology, and social acceptability. We don't want to be fooled by any one factor."

Once addicted, people manage their lives with varying degrees of success, according to the same combination of factors Henningfield mentions. They can operate normally for an indefinite period of time. Eventually, however, they start to slip, which is often the first time they become aware of their chemical dependence. By Kitty Dukakis's report, this is what happened to her; and she was smart enough to recognize what such a dependency meant right away because of her previous experience of an addiction slowly, quietly, and inexplicably taking over her life.

What Causes Headaches, and How Can I Cure Them?

"My brain is splitting in two." "It's like a vise on my skull." "I feel as if elephants were using my temple for a trampoline." Varied and often witty are the phrases over

Getting Off the Hook

In the case of alcohol and other powerful drugs, it's not easy to separate simple recreational use from addiction. If you can answer "yes" to several of the following questions (based on National Council on Alcoholism guidelines), you may need qualified medical help.

- *Do you occasionally feel guilty about drinking or using drugs?*
- *Does drinking or drug use frequently cause conflicts with others?*
- *Does drinking or drug use often upset your daily schedule?*
- *Do you often feel so mentally and physically down after drinking or drug use that you put off work or other obligations?*
- *Do you conceal or lie about your drinking or drug use?*
- *Do you find yourself consuming or stocking increasingly larger amounts of alcohol or drugs?*
- *Do you sometimes "binge" on alcohol or drugs? ("Binging" can be defined as consuming without stopping, pacing, or otherwise controlling yourself, even beyond the point at which you perceive a loss of control.)*
- *Do you eat little, irregularly, or poorly when drinking or using drugs?*
- *Do you sometimes experience memory loss during—or regarding—episodes of drinking or drug use?*

- *Do you tend to drink or use drugs to prepare yourself for certain kinds of tasks, experiences, or occasions?*
- *Do you often drink or use drugs when you're alone?*
- *Do you repeatedly find yourself unable to keep your own resolutions about controlling your drinking or drug use?*
- *Do you feel that people are treating you badly for no reason that you can understand?*

Addiction treatments vary widely according to the particular drug and drug-use history. The most successful treatments in general are self-help programs that feature repeated contact with people who can reinforce positive, nonaddictive behaviors and who can serve as watchdogs for mental, emotional, and physical problems that the addict can't—or won't—identify. Alcoholics Anonymous and Cocaine Anonymous are two model programs of this type. Contact national, state, and local public health services for confidential advice on programs and treatments for specific situations.

80 million Americans use to describe their headaches; but the discussion usually stops there. Few bother to find out what really lies behind the pain they feel. To them, "A headache is a headache." To brain researchers, there are many kinds of headaches: some that are merely nuisances and some that are important signals of danger in the brain, body, or life-style of the sufferer.

Medical science currently divides headaches into three broad categories: (1) tension headaches, (2) vascular headaches, and (3) headaches due to physical injury or disease. The categories do overlap somewhat. A single headache, for example, may begin as a tension headache and change into a migraine (or vascular) headache. Nevertheless, the categories are worth examining individually to demonstrate that a particular headache sensation may point to a distinct brand of headache, with its own characteristic causes, treatments, and implications.

Tension Headaches. The most common type of headache, the tension headache is triggered by muscle contraction resulting from situational stress or physical exertion. If anxiety causes you to hunch your shoulders, keep your neck stiff, or grind your teeth for an extended period of time, or if you tax your back muscles moving furniture, the strain may travel to the nerves in your brain, producing a constant pain with slight variations in intensity. For most people, the sensation is that of a tight band around the brain. It affects both sides of the head—most commonly in the front, but possibly on the top or back.

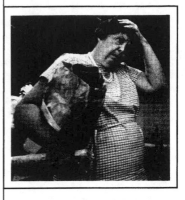

Muscular tension, often associated with a mentally or emotionally stressful situation, is the most common cause of a headache.

Tension headaches respond very well to nonprescription medications like aspirin, acetaminophen, and ibuprofen. It's also possible to get rid of them quickly and enjoyably by having someone massage the tense muscle group that seems to be responsible for the headache. Recurrent sufferers should consider incorporating into their daily regimen muscle-relaxing habits and breaks. Supposing your regular schedule involves a lot of paperwork and you frequently get headaches that build up as the day goes on, consider seeing an eye doctor. You may be overstraining the muscles around your eyes.

Vascular Headaches. For diagnostic purposes, doctors divide vascular headaches into four subcategories:

Migraine Headaches. These are the most debilitating headaches of all. The victim goes through several hours to several days of a prostrating pain that throbs with every heartbeat and is often accompanied by nausea and vomiting. Doctors used to believe that a migraine resulted from abnormally dilated blood vessels in the head, but in recent years they've discovered that the source of a migraine is a tidal wave of electrochemical activity in the brain, most frequently stirred up by stress, hunger, sen-

23

Types of Headaches

Tension Headache
cause: muscle contraction
symptom: pain on both sides of the head
cures: bed rest, massage, nonprescription drugs

Vascular Headache: Migraine
causes: stress, hunger, sensory overload, fatigue, hormone fluctuation, withdrawal
symptoms: prostrating pain on one side of the head, nausea, vomiting
cures: bed rest, possibly prescription drugs

Vascular Headache: Cluster
causes: same as for migraine
symptoms: slightly less pain than migraine, possibly stuffy sinus
cures: same as for migraine

Vascular Headache: Hypertensive
cause: high blood pressure
symptom: dull head pain
cure: bed rest

Vascular Headache: Toxic
causes: food or fume chemicals, allergies, changes in weather
symptoms: varying degrees of head pain
cures: withdrawal from cause, possibly prescription drugs

Headache Due to Injury/Disease
causes: infection, neurological problems, physical trauma, anemia
symptoms: head pain similar to or different from any of the other headaches, often accompanied by numbing, loss of balance, weakness
cure: medical attention to cause(s)

sory overload, fatigue, hormone fluctuations, or addiction withdrawal. Many migraine sufferers are forewarned of an attack by seeing spots, flashes, blank patches (either all-white or all-black), arcs, auras, or a zigzag pattern before their eyes. When the migraine finally strikes, it's almost always confined to one side of the head.

Treating a migraine headache is a complicated matter. People who are perfectionists or who place excessive demands upon their energies are more likely than the average person to have recurring migraines that resist therapy. A full-scale change in attitude and life-style may be the only answer. A tendency toward migraines can also be inherited. Assuming these factors are not relevant to you, then the odds are high that you won't suffer migraines at all. If you do, the only possible cure—short of riding it out in a dark, quiet bedroom—is a prescription-strength drug that can have a counteractive effect on your troubled brain chemistry. Among the medications that have proved most effective are ergotamine, methysergide, and verapamil.

Cluster Headaches. Cluster headaches are similar to migraines, but not as harsh. They're not pre-announced by visual light shows, they seldom cause nausea, and they don't stay around as long (usually two to three episodes in a single day, each episode lasting anywhere from ten minutes to a couple of hours). The single sensation that most distinguishes them from migraine headaches is a stuffy sinus. Otherwise, the cause and treatment factors are the same.

Hypertensive Headaches. As the name suggests, hypertensive headaches are occasioned by high blood pressure, which can make itself felt throughout the brain's circulatory system. The pain is dull and quickly relieved by bed rest. A check with a physician about high blood pressure is advisable.

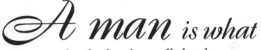

A man is what he thinks about all day long.
—Ralph Waldo Emerson

Toxic Headaches. These headaches are brewed by chemicals from food (prime culprits: cheese, chocolate, and citrus fruits) or fumes (such as carbon monoxide). They can also come from allergies and changes in the weather. Medical tests are frequently able to determine whether one's headaches are toxic and what can be done to avoid them.

Headaches Due to Physical Injury or Disease. The most insidious form of headache is the one that is caused by an undetected malady: a fever-producing infection in the sinuses, bloodstream, or lymph system; a neurological problem in the brain, ears, eyes, teeth, face, or spine; a trauma caused by a physical blow, tumor, or blood clot; or even a general state of anemia. Often this kind of headache has a discernibly different feeling than a normal tension headache, but just as often it doesn't. Headaches that are especially severe or that are attended by numbness, loss of balance, or sensations of weakness are always suspect. If you're concerned about an unusual headache symptom or about a new pattern of headaches in your life, don't hesitate to seek professional advice.

SCHIZO-PHRENICS

WHAT GOES ON IN THEIR MINDS?

Sometime early in adolescence we decide that a "schizo" is an individual with a split personality: Dr. Jekyll and Mr. Hyde, Bruce Wayne and Batman, the sweet girl next door who gossips behind people's backs, the honor student who secretly tortures cats. The true nature of schizophrenia is vastly different and infinitely more complicated, for the "split" in a schizophrenic's mind is not between two opposing personalities but between a single personality's thoughts and emotions.

At its worst, schizophrenia is the most severe and multifaceted form of mental illness: classic madness in the popular imagination. Estimating solely on the basis of reported cases, statisticians tell us that full-blown schizophrenia affects about 2 percent of the world's population. But the condition is so apt to be misreported—or not reported at all—that the real percentage of victims is almost certainly much higher, not to mention the additional percentage of people who suffer milder forms of schizophrenia.

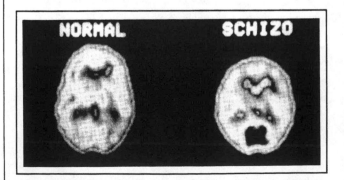

The PET scan on the left shows the glucose consumption activity of a normal brain; the one on the right shows the glucose consumption activity of a schizophrenic brain (see page 30 for more information on PET scans).

If schizophrenics are not split personalities (strictly speaking), then what are they? Consider "Lewis," a textbook case. At the age of twenty-two, Lewis was just beginning his career as an electrician when he began having episodes of profound distraction. Forgetting his work, he would brood for hours at a time. These ruminations ultimately took the form of hearing voices, and from these voices he developed the notion that he knew things no one else knew and, therefore, had a unique mission in life. Exactly what this knowledge or this mission was, he could never quite understand or articulate, but his feeling of being different from all other people gradually made him unable to conduct a normal life. He became paranoid regarding imaginary enemies, whose voices he could also hear. He turned apathetic during situations that he deemed irrelevant to his mission and violent whenever he encountered what he considered to be threats to his mission.

Although he lacked any clear picture of the mystery besieging him, Lewis's moment-by-moment fantasies were often very intricate and precise. Once he was standing at

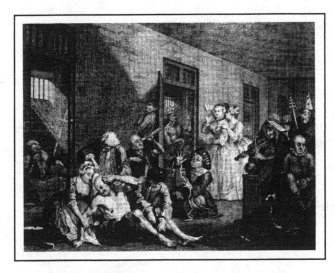

As late as the eighteenth century, schizophrenia and other forms of mental illness were considered beastly behaviors, and victims were treated like animals in cages. As shown in this drawing by the English artist William Hogarth of the notorious Bedlam Hospital in London, patients were routinely kept in chains and visited by curiosity seekers.

a busy intersection waiting for the light to change when he overheard a conversation next to him about butter. At the same moment a truck went by bearing the logo "Bond Bread." Convinced that the simultaneity of "bread" and "butter" was a fatefully prearranged signal that he was in serious immediate danger from his enemies, Lewis fled to a park bench, the nearest quiet, private, and, therefore, "safe" spot.

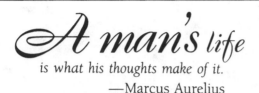

is what his thoughts make of it.
—Marcus Aurelius

Lewis's particular case history may be idiosyncratic, but his general mental condition falls into a well-established pattern. From anonymous bag ladies who scream at invisible assailants to the notorious psychotic John W. Hinckley, who shot President Reagan to impress film star Jodie Foster, all schizophrenics tend to exhibit the same characteristics: preoccupation, disordered thoughts and statements, auditory hallucinations, and delusions. The line separating what schizophrenics imagine from what they actually experience disappears, and so does their control over the behavior that issues from this confusion.

Schizophrenia seems to result from irregularities in the workings of dopamine, a neurochemical that facilitates message transmission among brain cells. As often happens, science stumbled upon the cause by trying out every conceivable cure. A century ago, German manufacturers synthesized a group of new dyes chemically called phenothiazines. Because a similar group of dyes had proved effective in treating malaria, doctors began experimenting to see if phenothiazines might be good for treating anything. By the early 1950s, French doctors had established that a phenothiazine known as chlorpromazine was remarkably effective in taming the worst symptoms of schizophrenia. Working backward from the logical conclusion that schizophrenia was a chemical disorder, researchers established a connection between dopamine problems in the brain and schizophrenia in the mind. They went on to produce an even more therapeutic drug, haloperidol; and thus, in the second half of the 1950s, history witnessed a dramatic reduction in the total number of institutionalized mental patients.

Regrettably, neither chlorpromazine nor haloperidol is a full-fledged cure for schizophrenia. Nor is the search for possible causes of schizophrenia over, despite what science has learned about dopamine irregularities. Recent genetic studies have shown that heredity can also play a role in the development of schizophrenia. So can stressful environmental factors (which, after all, contribute to the onset and progress of virtually any illness—mental or physical). Some doctors speculate that the initial catalyst for schizophrenia may be a viral infection in the brain. If this is true, a protective vaccine may someday be possible.

When I examined myself and my methods of thought, I came to the conclusion that the gift of fantasy has meant more to me than my talent for absorbing positive knowledge.

—Albert Einstein

Most likely, schizophrenia has multiple causes, and the same is probably true for other types of brain malfunctioning that we call "madness." We've come a long way toward recognizing that serious mental aberrations are, in fact, illnesses and not personality problems or incidents of demonic possession. Nevertheless, we still have quite a way to go. Dr. Richard Restak, author of many popular and scientific books about the brain, warns, "Research into schizophrenia governs only a fraction of the money allotted to cancer, an illness that equals but does not exceed the cost of schizophrenia in terms of workdays lost, hospitalization, and costs of medicine."

In the fight to wipe out schizophrenia and other forms of mental illness, research dollars make sense, but there's a lot to be said for personal action as well. The more we learn about how the mind works for good or for bad, the better equipped we are to help ourselves and others live in a mad, mad world.

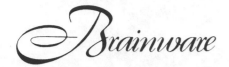

Brainware

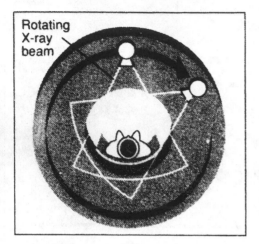

Computerized Axial Tomography Scanner
During the late 1960s and early 1970s, the invention of the Computerized Axial Tomography scanner, or CAT scan, literally turned the treatment of brain disease on its head. Doctors can now use the device to obtain crisp layer-by-layer, angle-by-angle photographs of any tissue damage or tumors in the brain's interior. The patient lies down on a table with his or her head inserted into the hole of a doughnut-shaped scanner. Inside this scanner moves an X-ray tube, passing beams through the brain as it rotates. A computer renders these beams into "slice images" of the brain that show varying physical densities in shades of black and white. Thus, doctors have a map of the brain from which they can determine precisely the size and configuration of structural irregularities.

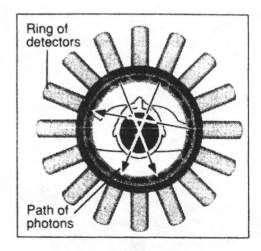

Positron Emission Tomography Scanner
Although the CAT scan makes it possible for doctors to see the inside of the brain, it doesn't show them how the brain is functioning. The Positron Emission Tomography scanner, or PET scan, does. Since its 1976 debut, the PET scan has stunned the scientific community with glowing, multihued, step-by-step pictures of the brain's chemical activity. First the patient is injected with a very low-level radioactive dye. Then his or her head is surrounded with a ring of 160 radiation detectors. These detectors translate different brain chemicals into different colors, which are then projected onto a screen. The real beauty of the PET scan is that it can photograph mental illness as well as physical illness. The brains of schizophrenics or manic-depressives, for example, can be instantly identified with a PET scan because the colors reveal distinctive abnormalities in glucose consumption that attend these disorders.

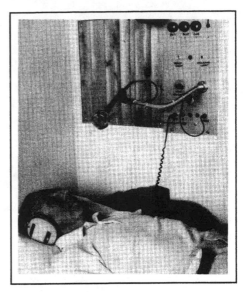

Recorded brain-wave pattern before using Hemi-Sync.

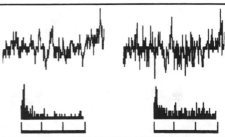

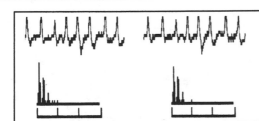

Recorded brain-wave pattern after using Hemi-Sync.

Hemi-Sync

Coming from another mind culture altogether, the Hemi-Sync is a stereo headset and sound system designed to elicit better right brain/left brain coordination. It's the mid-1980s brainchild of Robert Monroe, the chief guru of the "out-of-body experience," whereby an individual learns to be conscious from a perspective outside his or her physical body (something that often appears to happen in dreams). The Hemi-Sync is not necessarily intended to transport the user beyond his or her flesh; instead, it's meant to induce a state of consciousness that is eminently open to suggestion and self-tutoring. Pulsing tones of different frequencies are sent to each ear, and ultimately the user's brain waves assume a slow-wave Delta rhythm. In this manner, the two hemispheres are transformed into a state of deep sleep—the Delta state—and yet the user remains fully awake. Based on tests at the Menninger Foundation in Topeka, Kansas, the ensuing bi-hemispheric mental activity is akin to that of a Zen master. Once the user achieves this state, he or she may choose to plug in a subliminal self-help tape. Theoretically, it's the best right/left time for it.

2
CONSCIOUSNESS

rove you exist. It's a challenge that
bedevils anyone who speculates
about life, from grade-school wise
guys to doctors of philosophy. The
seventeenth-century intellectual René
Descartes, with a characteristically French
tidy-mindedness, insisted, "I think, therefore
I am." For most of us, however, thinking is
not the full-time job it was for Descartes. It's
enough for us to say that we *know* we exist—
the proof lies in the fact that we are *conscious*
beings. But what is consciousness? It seems
so obvious, and yet it is the single most baffling phenomenon associated with the human
brain.

In everyday language, we associate "consciousness" with "awareness" and describe it
as if it were some sort of light on a dimmer

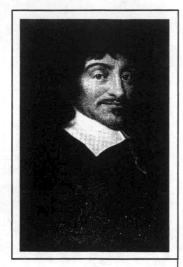

René Descartes

switch: It's either "off" or "on," and its "on" state has various possible degrees of intensity. In fact, consciousness is more like a sea of ever-shifting currents. We can exercise all our mental faculties on a tricky analytical problem and at the same time be oblivious to our surroundings (the condition of "absentmindedness"). We can be driving our car smoothly and safely along a familiar route; and yet our minds can wander so far away that when we're forced to make an unexpected stop, we realize we've lost complete track of the previous half-hour (the so-called "time-gap experience"). Under severe mental or physical pressure—such as witnessing the death of a mate or suffering a broken limb—our attention can focus with clarity on situational problems and simultaneously block out whatever threatens to disturb our sanity (the medical state known as "shock").

A much more mundane evasion of the reality around us is the common daydream, which enters into all of our waking lives, voluntarily and involuntarily, several times a day. Although the word "daydreaming" has acquired a negative connotation in our action-oriented culture, experts are now claiming that such moments of self-absorption can have both practical and psychological value. Certainly some daydreams can be neurotic and counterproductive, but more often these creative fantasies are sources of refreshment, pleasure, and/or inspiration. The same can be said about our night-dreaming, which, like sleeping in general, is simply another form of consciousness.

Although the phrase is embedded in the language, we really never "lose" consciousness. Even a person who faints, suffers a prostrating blow to the head, or lapses into a coma retains some form of consciousness or, as the famed psychologist Julian Jaynes prefers to call it, "reactivity." It's more accurate to think of these alleged "unconscious" situations as *shifts* in consciousness, causing the brain to filter experience in a different manner.

Every second, 100 million messages from our nervous system bombard our brain. Only several hundred are permitted above our brain stem, and only a few of these receive some sort of response. One possible response may be the type of awareness that can be translated directly and immediately into words, whether we're "talking" to

ourselves or communicating with others. An alternative
response may be an action that doesn't include such an
awareness: This action could be anything from sleepwalk-
ing to a skill as seemingly "aware" as playing a complicated piano sonata, which would be impossible if the
mind of the player consciously registered the movement
of every single finger muscle. Yet another possible response may be a mental or physiological event that is
strictly internal—one that eludes "rational" self-perception
and doesn't trigger any observable action.

In *Doors of Perception,* Aldous Huxley referred to the
mechanism that filters our sensory experience as "the reducing valve." We use it to screen things that we don't
need—or choose—to focus on for our immediate survival. Huxley took mes-
caline (an hallucinogen
derived from cactus
buds) as a quick means
of opening this valve
and experiencing the
unconventional varieties
of consciousness that
mystics describe. In
doing so, he was acting
out a desire that is
probably innate in the
human psyche. Psychol-
ogist Andrew Weil
notes in *Natural Mind,*
"Anyone who watches

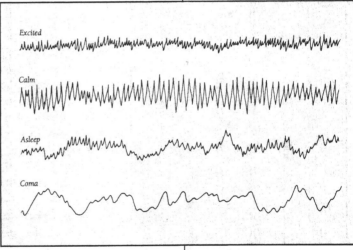

very young children will find them regularly practicing
techniques that induce striking changes in mental states.
Three- and four-year-olds commonly whirl themselves
into stupors. They hyperventilate and have other children
squeeze them around the chest until they feel faint."
Among other activities, adults turn to aerobics, long-distance running, dancing, sex, skydiving, and even religious
ritual for the same purpose.

These brain-wave variations capture different grada-
tions of attention: excited, calm, asleep, and coma.

Like Huxley, they also turn to drugs. Alcohol and tobacco continue to be the mind-benders of choice, but as a
legacy of the soul-searching 1960s, there is also widespread experimentation with psychoactive chemical compounds like marijuana, lysergic acid diethylamide (LSD),

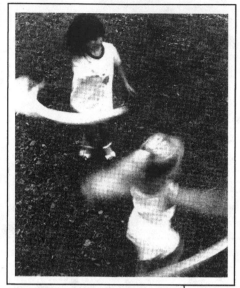

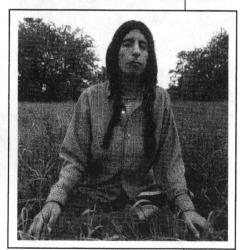

Children have their own, natural ways of seeking altered states of consciousness.

A purist in the Eastern meditative arts assumes the traditional lotus position, with each foot placed astride the opposite knee. It can take months of limbering exercises with supportive pillows before this position is comfortable, but once you master the position, it gives your spinal column ideal support and helps you to remain balanced in repose.

amphetamines, barbiturates, cocaine, heroin, and nitrous oxide ("laughing gas"). Unfortunately, this experimentation can easily turn into addiction, in which case any benefits derived from apprehending reality in new ways are overshadowed by the mind-owner's increasing loss of self-control and physical health.

There remains, however, a positive side to the 1960s' exploration of counter-consciousness. It taught Western civilization that the mind has more possibilities than our ordinary modes of consciousness can imagine and, consequently, that life has more possibilities than our ordinary daily experience allows. As we move into an era that promises to be far more demanding of our individual spirits, emotions, and intellects, we will need to tap those possibilities more efficiently and effectively. The better we understand the many forms that consciousness can take, the better we can apply that understanding to enhance the quality of our lives.

In this chapter, you will learn more about the rhythmical shifts in consciousness that are programmed into the daily life of your brain via your "body clock." Left to its natural self, it is this body clock that determines when we're the most wide-awake and when we're the most sleepy. If we ignore this timing mechanism or tamper with it, we inevitably suffer. If we cooperate with it, we inevitably function more pleasurably and more productively. You will find out, for example, how to combat jet lag and disruptive work schedule changes and how to derive more satisfaction from the dreaming activity that your brain conducts regularly each night, whether your daytime consciousness knows it or not.

You will also examine what authorities like Sigmund Freud and Carl Jung have to say about how the intrinsic organization of our mind's consciousness processes and shapes our personalities. And you will discover ways in which you can create states of consciousness that are desirable (for example, more peaceful or more energized)

Peace of Mind: Eastern Style

Of all possible states of consciousness, none is more sought after than peace of mind. In Eastern cultures, this quest gave rise to the art of meditation. Essentially, meditation involves striving to achieve tranquility, patience, and clear-headedness by learning to immerse yourself in a single mental task, such as visualizing a particular image, or contemplating a particular word-sound, or even attending to your breath. The effect of meditation on the brain is a slowing and deepening of the brain-wave pattern from Beta to Alpha or (in advanced stages) even Theta, which produces a mildly altered state of consciousness akin to mysticism (for more about brain waves, see Chapter I, "How the Brain Works").

While developing adeptness at meditation requires time and qualified direction, you can begin to get a sense of what meditation feels like after you've been practicing the following exercise for one or two weeks:

• Sit comfortably with your eyes closed in a place where you won't be disturbed.

• Focus your awareness on breathing from your diaphragm, just below your stomach. Feel your breathing and concentrate solely on it.

• After a couple of minutes, begin counting each exhalation, starting with one and proceeding up through ten and then repeating the process, again and again. If you lose track of the count, gently draw your concentration back to your breathing and resume the count at one.

• After approximately seven to ten minutes, stop counting and simply feel your breathing for a few more minutes. Then gently return your mind to the everyday world.

and counteract those that are not (like having insomnia or a hangover). Finally, you will come to understand more about such mysterious yet potentially practical phenomena of consciousness as hypnosis, subliminal perception, and the type of mental dissociation that manifests itself in multiple personality disorder.

Why Is My Brain Usually More Alert at Some Times of the Day than Others?

Different people swear by different preventive remedies. Evangelist Billy Graham does deep-breathing exercises. Geraldine Ferraro, 1984 Democratic vice-presidential candidate, goes on an all-day fast. Actor Michael York has arguably the most inscrutable cure: He wears cut-up brown paper bags in his shoes. What they are all trying to avoid is "jet lag," a syndrome of weariness and disorientation

that often plagues long-distance air travelers who are
forced to cope with a radically altered day-and-night pattern in a relatively short period of time.

What jet lag makes us realize is that the human mind
(in harmony with the body) is subject to an inner clock, a
rhythmic pattern of alertness and fatigue analogous to the
daily cycle. Placed in an artificial environment where
there are no day-and-night cues, most humans will settle
into a roughly twenty-five-hour pattern of activity and
rest. Others, however, will function in forty-eight- to fifty-
four-hour cycles—remaining awake and active for thirty-
three to thirty-six hours and resting for twelve to fifteen
hours. Either way, we all make some internal compromises in adjusting to the day-and-night cycle of the local
outside environment.

Within the course of a "real-world" day, energy cycles
can vary greatly from individual to individual. Usually,
these variances correlate with the individual's personality
and engrained body-temperature pattern. People who are
early risers by nature and function best in the morning
(nicknamed "larks" by behavioral scientists) tend to have
a slightly higher body temperature in the morning—any
fraction up to one degree Fahrenheit—which results in
better mental performance. For unknown reasons, they
also tend to be introverted. So-called "owls," or night
people, have a higher temperature in the evening hours
and are generally more extroverted (again, for unknown
reasons).

Regardless of whether you're a lark or an owl, you'll experience a midday dip in energy and you'll have your
own ninety-minute cycles of mental acuity versus listless-
ness, and hunger versus no hunger, throughout the day,
continuing even when you're asleep, in which case mental
acuity and possibly hunger are manifested in dreams.
Stimulants and/or sedatives may set you free from these
built-in cycles for a few hours, but you pay a stiff price
for the freedom. Sooner or later you must return to your
natural schedule, and the trip back is sure to be rougher
the longer or the farther you've been away.

A much more serious disturbance to a human being's
inner clock than long-distance jet travel is an abruptly altered or erratic work-life pattern. According to Dr.
Charles Czeisler of Harvard University and the Center for

Design of Industrial Schedules in Boston, Massachusetts, "A shiftwork schedule can wreak havoc on physiological timing systems that control the release of hormones, control the timing of when we sleep and when we wake, even control the timing of when we feel alert and when we feel ready for sleep." An individual's body-clock disturbances can be harmful to others as well. They've been officially blamed for airplane disasters, misjudgments in space probes, acts of medical malpractice, ship collisions, and even the March 28, 1979, near-disaster at the Three Mile Island nuclear plant, which occurred at 4:00 A.M. and involved new members of the graveyard shift.

What can be done to make body-clock transitions less uncomfortable and dangerous? For shiftworkers (a population in America that includes one out of every four men and one out of every six women), the answer is to lengthen the schedule of rotations, so that a given worker stays on the same shift for a longer period of time. Shifts should also be altered on a one-step basis whenever possible; for example, a worker who is accustomed to an 8:00-to-4:00 schedule should be transferred next to a 4:00-to-12:00 schedule and not to a 12:00-to-8:00 schedule. Finally, shiftworkers need to begin gradually changing their daily schedule in advance of a shift change, so it is less disruptive of their lives when it comes.

Suppose you have to transfer from an 8:00-to-4:00 schedule to a 4:00-to-12:00 schedule. Since it takes approximately a week to make a minimally acceptable adjustment to an eight-hour schedule change, you can start a week ahead of time to nudge your eating and sleeping times closer to the times you will be eating and sleeping after the change. It may be logistically impossible to make a full transition ahead of time, but any change in the right direction that you can manage will be beneficial. It's also a good idea to avoid stressful situations, substance abuse, or other types of physical and mental overextension during at least the week before and the week after the change.

In the case of jet lag, the same logic applies. Suppose you are planning to fly from your home in New York to London. It takes approximately three days to recover from a five-hour time-zone change, so three days prior to your flight, you may want to begin gradually changing the

New York

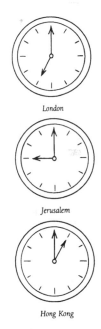

London

Jerusalem

Hong Kong

Experts in jet lag say it takes three days to recover from a five-hour time difference (for example, traveling from New York to London); four days to recover from a seven-hour time difference (from New York to Jerusalem); and five days to recover from an eleven-hour time difference (from New York to Hong Kong).

times you eat and sleep so they will correspond more
closely to the times you will be eating and sleeping in England. Some soon-to-be travelers find that eating five or
six small meals during the day, rather than the normal
three at the normal three times, works wonders. So does
taking a nap during the day to supplement shorter night-
time sleep.

As a last resort, don't entirely dismiss Michael York's
mysterious paper-bag cure. Presumably, he relies on this
strange custom to remind himself that he's going through
a time change. Experts in consciousness claim that anything keeping you mindful of the jet-lag problem—
whether it's wearing cut-up paper in your shoes or a special charm around your neck—can possibly help you to
psych it out.

Are There Foods I Can Eat to Calm Down or Pep Up?

Pacing the floor? Grinding your teeth? Beating your head
against the wall? Quick! Grab a candy bar! Chances are
that by the time you're licking your fingers, you'll wonder
how in the world you got so upset.

According to Dr. Richard Wurtman, Dr. Judith Wurtman, and Dr. John Fernstrom of the Massachusetts Institute of Technology, a candy bar loaded with carbohydrates
can, in fact, be an anxiety antidote. Their experiments
have demonstrated how substances in ordinary edibles
can effect changes in our brain's chemistry and, consequently, alter the way we feel, think, and behave.

When you eat a candy bar, for example, the sugar (a
carbohydrate) enters your bloodstream quickly and stimulates production of serotonin, a chemical transmitter in
the brain. Serotonin relaxes you and, at least temporarily,
puts you in a better frame of mind to cope with life's
daily challenges and aggravations. That's possibly one reason why President Reagan always kept a bowl of jelly
beans on the table at cabinet meetings!

The logic behind the candy cure is short and sweet.
Chief among all brain nutrients are two amino acids, tyrosine and tryptophan, that work to counterbalance each
other. The brain metabolizes tyrosine, which is present in

high-protein foods, into two different neurotransmitters, norepinephrine and dopamine. These neurotransmitters sharpen your conscious awareness, increase your attention span, and even help your brain to perform rational functions more efficiently. Sometimes, however, they can put you into overdrive, getting you so hyped up that you can't handle opposition or setbacks.

By contrast, tryptophan, the amino acid present in high-carbohydrate foods, stimulates the production of serotonin—nature's remedy for both red-hot anger and the moody blues. Besides making you calm, serotonin enables you to withstand pain and discomfort by raising your level of endorphins (the brain's natural pain-killing chemicals). Increased serotonin also helps you to conquer insomnia. Wurtman, Wurtman, and Fernstrom are now studying whether tryptophan supplements can be used to assuage chronic pain or even the extreme pain associated with life-threatening diseases like cancer.

If you want to boost your mental energies for an important meeting or test, scientists recommend a natural dose of tyrosine, via small portions of relatively high-protein foods like fish, shellfish, skinless chicken, low-fat cottage cheese, tofu, or skim milk. Heavy meals and fat-laden foods require more time to digest. This, in turn, keeps blood in the stomach area and away from the brain, which makes it harder for you to concentrate.

On the other hand, when you feel the need to proceed through life in a more well-tempered manner—or to enjoy a smoother path to sleep—carbohydrates, not proteins, will help you jack up your serotonin level. A candy bar, though, is not the only solution. Despite the candy bar's attractive packaging and gut appeal, a simple apple, potato, bagel, bran muffin, or small helping of rice will do the trick. If the candy bar you favor contains protein-rich nuts, it can even be counterproductive, since combining carbohydrates and proteins sometimes inhibits serotonin production altogether.

Whatever your preference, it makes sense to stash the best of both types of foods within convenient reach at home and at work. Candy counters may be on every block, and candy bars may be alluringly pocket-sized, but a 200-calorie bagel will soothe your weight-consciousness far better than a 500-calorie Baby Ruth.

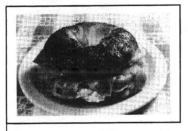

Sorry! Delicious as a bagel with lox can be, the calming effects of the high-carbohydrate bread are canceled out by the energizing effects of the high-protein salmon.

THE FLOW

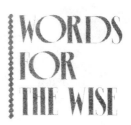

The expression "go with the flow" arose in the 1960s to describe a passive, hassle-free yielding to the circumstances around you. Psychologist Mihaly Csikszentmihalyi (pronounced "chik-SENT-me-high-yee") meant something quite different when he announced his flow theory in the 1970s. The flow, as he describes it, is a state of intense concentration akin to ecstasy. And it's a purely natural state, one that no drug, diet, or device can duplicate. While it lasts, it's not only enjoyable, it also improves one's mental and physical performance.

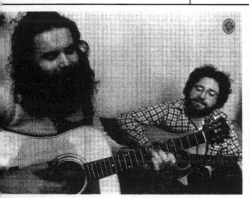

Rock climbers experience the flow when they're so involved in their task that they feel at one with the cliff face, incapable of falling. So do chess masters absorbed in a challenging match, in which case both players often lose all perception of time. And so do concert violinists in performance, if they get so wrapped up in their music that they sense they're producing it automatically. The most conversant with the flow experience, however, are young children. When we were preschool-age, we could often devote ourselves entirely to our made-up games and play effortlessly and joyfully for hours. As we matured, we became less and less inclined to yield ourselves so completely to any single activity.

Now Csikszentmihalyi argues that we can still achieve that wondrous, childlike sensation of clarity, purpose, and smooth-functioning during our adult years. It comes spontaneously if the activity at hand and the performer's skills are evenly matched—action merges with awareness, attention is completely centered, and the egoless performer winds up in complete control of what happens. "When you encounter challenges that are greater than your skills, that's anxiety," he states. "When your skills exceed the challenges, that's boredom."

Regrettably, you can't just "will" yourself into the flow. One approach lies in putting yourself into different flow-creating work or play situations by improving your skill level to match the challenge, or by increasing or reducing the challenge to match your skill level. The best choice depends on the circumstances. If you're a bored assembly-line worker, for example, you may be able to realize the flow by conditioning yourself to perform your tasks twice as fast (which shouldn't be too difficult, given your present skill level and the repetitiveness of assembly-line routines). If you've mastered swimming laps and want to make that activity more exhilarating, try executing your strokes as smoothly and gracefully as possible or stretching the total length of your swim. If you're having trouble sticking to an exercise regimen because it's too taxing, simplify it until you begin to enjoy it.

Another path to the flow involves making every effort to screen out distractions. When you're involved in a work or play activity, arrange matters so your environment will be pleasant, quiet, and free from interruption. Get as physically comfortable as possible. Stay mentally focused on the task at hand, gently returning your mind to that task whenever you sense your mind is wandering away. Eventually, you're likely to lapse into a spontaneous distraction-free state that is one of the primary catalysts of the flow.

Brain-wave studies at the University of Chicago indicate that the flow-state experience strongly resembles the meditative experience, which Csikszentmihalyi classifies as "the notion of learning to stop the world." One can never experience it on a full-time basis, he warns, but "if you cultivate the flow, you can have the experience several times a day, for minutes or even hours at a time."

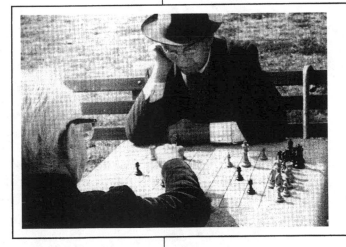

The flow state can be experienced no matter what kind of activity is involved—an emotive, artistic one, such as playing music, or a rational, logistic one, such as playing chess.

What Is Meant by My "Unconscious" or "Subconscious" Mind, and How Does It Affect My Life?

One might compare the relationship of the ego to the id with that between a rider and his horse. The horse provides the locomotor energy and the rider has the prerogative of determining the goal and of guiding the movements of his powerful mount toward it. But all too often in the relations between the ego and the id we find a picture of the less ideal situation in which the rider is obliged to guide his horse in the direction in which it itself wants to go.

—Sigmund Freud

Without a doubt, Sigmund Freud and Carl Jung are the two individuals who have had the most influence on how the twentieth century regards consciousness. In an effort to explain how we "know" more than we're actively aware of—either at any given moment or for virtually a lifetime—both men drew a simplistic but handy distinction between consciousness and unconsciousness (sometimes translated as "subconsciousness").

Freud maintained that our "unconscious mind" harbors all the bits of knowledge, memory, and intuition that we're not "consciously" attending to at the moment. Thus, the contents of the unconscious mind change somewhat as we shift our brain's attention to different things. The personality that emerges from Freud's conscious/unconscious mind has three dimensions: (1) the *superego,* which consists of all the behaviors, standards, and rules that are learned directly, or indirectly, from outside authorities; (2) the *ego,* which consists of the individual's innate powers of control, reason, judgment, and imagination; and (3) the *id,* which consists of the individual's raw emotions, impulses, and instincts.

The superego and the ego both have their "conscious" and "unconscious" elements, but the id is strictly unconscious—kept repressed by the superego and the ego. Every now and then, however, a small bit of unconscious data can unexpectedly spring full-blown into consciousness. Such is the stuff of madness and dreams, and the stuff of those amusing but embarrassingly revealing instances of misspeaking known as "Freudian slips"—saying "I'd like you to beat my boss," for example, instead of "I'd like you to meet my boss."

In Freud's view, the superego, the ego, and the id often come in conflict with each other, reacting to pressures emanating from the unconscious mind. Freudian psychotherapy involves exploring what the patient has "relegated" to the unconscious, out of forgetfulness, fear, shame, or anxiety. Much, if not all, of this relegated matter is presumed to be sexual in nature—as befits a theory forged in Victorian times.

Carl Jung was a disciple of Freud's, but broke from him on several key points. Like Freud, he retained the notion of a conscious mind and an unconscious mind for simplicity's sake, but he split the "unconscious mind" into two categories: (1) an ever-shifting "personal unconscious," consisting of details and issues in our own lives that we're not consciously attending, and (2) a stable "collective unconscious," consisting of patterns, images, and issues that are common to all humans and that shape how we reason, imagine, and live.

The personality that emerges from Jung's conscious/unconscious mind has three major dimensions: (1) a *persona,* which is the face that the individual presents to the outside world; (2) a *self,* which is the individual's "true" identity; and (3) an *anima* (for a male) or an *animus* (for a female), which is the individual's "soul-self," a force embedded in the unconscious mind with which the individual craves union. The anima/animus is

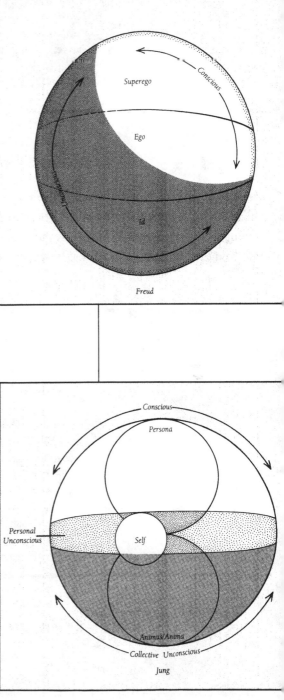

Freud

Jung

conceived as a sexual opposite (female for a male, male for a female) because of the yearning element involved in this soul-seeking, and, according to Jung, it plays a strong role in the individual's creative urge and search for a life-mate.

In Jung's view, inner conflicts occur when the various dimensions of the personality are not in harmony with each other. While the Freudian therapist focuses primarily on relieving the pressures imposed by a troublesome "unconscious" mind, the goal for a Jungian therapist is to assist clients to realize their "unconscious" potential—a balance of nature and spirit.

One of Jung's most intriguing theories involves what he labels "synchronicity"—the oddly coincidental occurrence of related images and/or events in our real-life experience during the same brief time period (for example, reading about pirates in the morning, overhearing a conversation about pirates that afternoon, and noting a window display of pirate mannequins that night). In Jungian terms, many of these seemingly fortuitous coincidences may, in fact, be engineered by forces at work on both a personal level and a collective unconscious level.

The most important single contribution made by pioneer psychologists like Freud and Jung is that they taught us to respect the possibility that everything we think, say, do, or experience—no matter how apparently trivial or accidental—has meaning. Even slips of the tongue and funny coincidences can lead us to know more about ourselves and others and how the human mind operates.

The dynamic

principle of fantasy is play, which belongs also to the child, and . . . appears to be inconsistent with the principle of serious work. But without this playing with fantasy, no creative work has ever yet come to birth.

—Carl Jung

Inspiration

is the impact of a fact on a well-prepared mind.
—Louis Pasteur

16

MULTIPLES

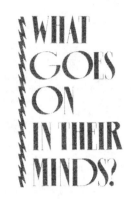

WHAT GOES ON IN THEIR MINDS?

Have you ever fantasized about having a secret twin who could replace you when you were tired, sick, scared, or faced with a burdensome task? Each year, the wish becomes so overpowering for an estimated 16,000 abused children in the United States that their minds somehow split into separate personalities. Victims of multiple personality disorder (MPD) or "multiples," their tormented brains generate anywhere from 8 to 180 competing personalities by adulthood, when the wish has long since turned into a curse.

What amazes scientists about multiples is that their alternate personalities behave as if they were fully autonomous people. Individual personalities master distinctive physical, intellectual, and interpersonal skills and develop different self-images relating to age, sex, physiognomy, life history, and belief systems. They also vary dramatically in posture, voice, handedness, and even such physiological features as brain-wave pattern, sensory acuity, immune system status, skin electrical response, pain threshold, allergic reaction, and healing rate.

How does the brain of a multiple effect these startling changes? We don't have a clue. All we know is that a given personality either steps in automatically to control the host body when an outside development calls for his or her special talents (a "responsive takeover") or else that personality simply usurps the host body when he

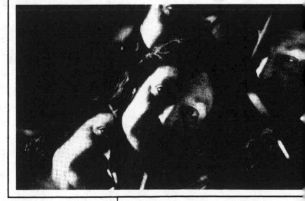

A multiple is not someone who has different, even opposite aspects contained within a single identity, but rather someone who has distinctly separate identities that may or may not know about each other.

or she feels like it (an "attack takeover"). Whether or not different personalities inhabit different parts of the brain or different streams of consciousness remains to be proven.

Billy Mulligan, described by Daniel Keyes in *The Minds of Billy Mulligan,* was born in 1955. During his childhood, he was sexually abused by his stepfather on a regular

From Outer Space to Inner Space

The Institute of Noetic Sciences is a nonprofit foundation designed to disseminate information about the mind among the public in general and among members of the scientific community and the helping professions in particular. Based in Sausalito, California, it was founded in 1973 with the help of Apollo 14 astronaut Edgar Mitchell, who conducted several in-space psychic communication experiments with a colleague back on Earth. In 1984, the Institute of Noetic Sciences held one of the largest seminars on multiple personality disorder ever held in this country. Pictured here is the masthead of the institute's newsletter, Investigations.

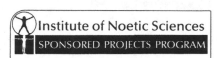

Institute of Noetic Sciences
SPONSORED PROJECTS PROGRAM

The Institute of Noetic Sciences was founded in 1973 by Dr. Edgar D. Mitchell, Apollo 14 astronaut, to support research and educational programs to expand mankind's understanding of the nature of consciousness and the mind-body link. Over the years, the Institute has funded a broad range of activities. The programs listed reflect the variety of our interests and our overall policy—to fund on a cost-effective basis those programs which will contribute to a better understanding of the inner person and universal consciousness.

basis (childhood sexual abuse is in the history of over 97 percent of multiples). By the time he was in his mid-twenties, he had spawned twenty-four different personalities. They include Christene [sic], an affectionate and artistic child; Ragen, an expert in munitions and karate who functions as a protector and who writes and speaks Serbo-Croatian; Arthur, an intellectual pacifist who talks with a British accent; and Adalana, an introverted teenage lesbian whose eyes twitch with nystagmus—an involuntary oscillation.

In therapy, several of Mulligan's personalities referred to being in control of the body as being "on the spot." One personality lucky enough to know about the others explained, "It's a big white spotlight. Everybody stands around it, watching or sleeping in their beds. And whoever steps on the spot is out in the world . . . whoever holds the spot holds the consciousness." Prior to therapy, most of Mulligan's personalities remained ignorant of many—or all—of the other personalities, so that their individual "conscious" lives were full of memory gaps, surprise predicaments, and desperately furtive coping strategies. As with most multiples, therapy couldn't meld Mulligan's personalities into one. It could only make them aware of each other so that they can now live together more harmoniously.

Therapists who work with multiples have been struck by how swiftly and cleanly their wounds heal and how fast they recover from colds or flu, compared to nonmultiples. Perhaps, suggests Brendan O'Regan of the Institute of Noetic Sciences (*noesis* is Greek for "intelligence"), this acceleration results from one personality concentrating on healing and nothing else. Speaking of research into how multiples function, O'Regan claims, "The benefits could be enormous in terms of our understanding of not only how mind and body are linked, but also in terms of psychosomatic medicine as a whole."

In fact, studies of multiples may hint at altogether new ways of programming our brains. For all the confusion they can stir up, a multiple's personalities occasionally display enviable cooperation. For example, an inebriated personality can "switch," voluntarily or involuntarily, to any one of a number of qualified personalities sober enough to drive a car. Several personalities can even engage in "parallel processing": for example, one may build a bookcase while others, separately and simultaneously, perform healing visualizations, plan dinner, and review French verbs. If science could determine how "switching" and "parallel processing" mechanisms work in the brains of multiples, could nonmultiples eventually be trained to make exclusively healthy, constructive use of dissociative states? No one knows yet.

Dr. John Kihlstrom offers guarded support for such a possibility in an essay in *The Unconscious Reconsidered,* an anthology edited by Dr. Kenneth Bowers and Dr. Donald Meichenbaum. "All of us appear to have the capacity to dissociate [i.e., 'compartmentalize' our minds], as in the case of dreams and other aspects of sleep," Kihlstrom admits. "At the same time, some of us are more prone to dissociate than others, and some of us have more voluntary control over dissociative processes, an attribute that may differentiate hypnotic virtuosos from the rest of the population." In theory, this means that some of us (and in time possibly all of us) may be able to train our minds to occasion and control the development of different personalities all using the same brain—a positive and constructive counterpart to the nightmare of involuntary, trauma-induced MPD.

Whatever the specific results may be, no one questions the significance of MPD research itself. In the words of Dr. Frank W. Putnam, Jr., of the National Institute of Mental Health, "The study of multiple personalities has something to offer the rest of us in terms of control of the mind and the body. I think multiples may, in fact, be one of those experiments of nature that will tell us more about ourselves."

Why Does My Brain Dream, and How Can I Remember and Use My Dreams More Effectively?

In our nightly dreams, each of us leads a second life. It's a life that's often disturbing or confusing (and, as a result, easy to forget), mainly because it doesn't follow the logic of our waking world. And yet it's a life that can bring us all manner of fresh sensations, emotions, and ideas that are unattainable by the light of day.

Science has not yet established the cause or biological function of dreaming. Until this century, science didn't even address dreams, considering them to be in the same realm as hallucinations, demonic possessions, or divine revelations. Finally, in 1953, researchers at the University of Chicago proved that all human beings dream four or five times a night, in roughly ninety-minute cycles. The key to this proof was the discovery that human beings—and most other animals, for that matter—exhibit rapid eye movement (REM) while dreaming. In other words, our eyes follow the sights of our dream life just as they follow the sights of our waking life. By electronically monitoring the eye movements of sleeping volunteers and waking them whenever they registered REM activity, re-searchers were able to chart the brain's typical dreaming pattern, and to identify a distinct brain-wave type associ-ated with dreaming.

Regarding how and why the brain dreams, scientists have numerous theories but no answers. To one group, dreaming is the right brain talking to itself, after having listened to the left brain most of the day. To another group, dreaming is a type of "off-line processing," in which the brain discharges thoughts and feelings that are nonproductive by waking-life standards. A third group thinks of dreaming as the brain's imaginative and self-instructive play with significant issues and images from the dreamer's daytime experience. A fourth group considers dreaming to be the brain's attempt at making sense of the unguided "firings" of random neurons during sleep.

While we may not know the physiological cause or function of dreams, we do know a great deal about their effects. Dreams can force us to confront what we prefer to repress or ignore, but they can also satisfy our secret desires. They can make us doubt our most cherished beliefs, yet they can also solve mysteries and provide creative inspiration. Throughout the ages people have successfully used the following techniques to improve their dream recall, break unpleasant dream patterns, enhance the quality and content of their dreams, and benefit from the insights that their dreams have to offer.

Plan to Remember Your Dreams. A simple shift in attitude can work wonders. Tell yourself several times during the day, especially before you retire at night, that you intend to remember your dreams. You may want to place an object with a scent—such as a bag of herbs, a sachet, or a room deodorant—near your bed as a "dream in-

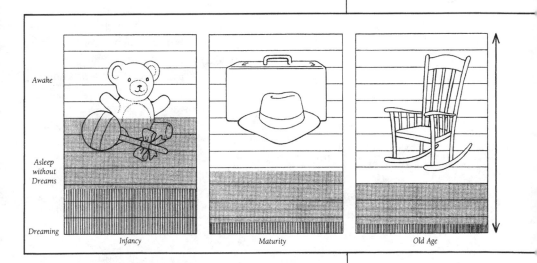

| | Infancy | Maturity | Old Age |

Awake

Asleep without Dreams

Dreaming

An infant (less than one year old) passes approximately forty percent of his or her fourteen sleeping hours in dreams. An adult around twenty-one to sixty-five years old dreams about twenty percent of his or her seven to eight sleeping hours. Beyond the age of seventy, an individual usually sleeps around six hours, but the percentage of dreamtime remains the same.

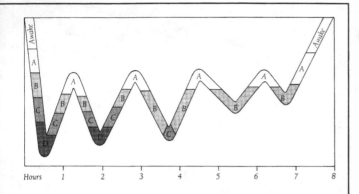

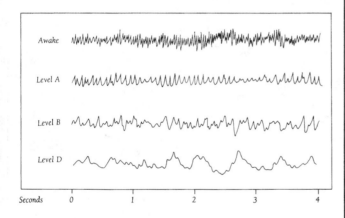

In a typical eight-hour night's sleep, we go through four levels of sleeping consciousness, with Level D being the deepest sleep. The first time we return to Level A sleep after having descended to Level D sleep (usually after ninety minutes), we dream. This cycle repeats itself four more times, with four more dreaming periods. The brain produces characteristic brain waves at Levels A, B, and D.

ducer," so that you are subliminally influenced to think about your dreams and to remember them when you awake. Whatever you do, lie still for a moment after awakening and concentrate on recalling your dreams. Ask yourself, "How do I feel?" or "What am I thinking about?" Often these open-ended questions will ultimately lead you back to key dream images.

Record Your Dreams and Ponder Them. Keep a dream journal and make individual entries in it as soon as possible after you've had a dream. Review each dream after you've recorded it. Note any images or feelings that seem to relate to images or feelings in your waking life. Avoid rushing to interpret the meaning of a dream and stick to your own intuitions and judgments rather than to those of an outside source (your dream about an ocean, for instance, might mean something entirely different from someone else's dream about an ocean). After you've accumulated several dreams in your journal, look for recurring patterns of images and feelings. Ask yourself, "Why am I confronted with these images and feelings at this point in my life?"

Experiment with Your Dream Life. If you have a problem to solve or a creative challenge of any kind in your waking life, you may want to tackle it in your dreams through an age-old technique known as "incubating a

Night School

The famous English poet and engraver William Blake drew much of his artistic inspiration from dreams. He also had one of the most celebrated problem-solving dreams in history. One night he dreamed that his beloved brother, long dead, recited a protocol for producing engravings more effectively and efficiently. When he woke up, he remembered the protocol, tested it, and the result was a revolutionary new engraving process. This particular Blake engraving depicts a more troublesome episode in the history of dreams: the Biblical Job tormented by nightmares.

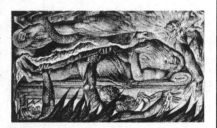

dream." Several times during the day, and especially before sleeping, tell yourself that you want to dream about a certain subject. The next morning, lie in bed and make an effort to recall your dream. Record it as soon as possible, whether or not it seems to be a response to your incubated intention. Review the dream several times over the next few days to see if you can establish any connection. You may be lucky with incubation right away, but most likely it will take repeated practice to work.

Another, more complicated dream experiment is to try "lucid dreaming"—becoming aware that you are dreaming *while* you are dreaming and perhaps even influencing the content of your dream as it goes along. Tell yourself several times the day before that you intend to awake right after one of your dreams. When you do awake (either during the night or in the morning), concentrate on recalling and reliving your last dream. Then, as you prepare to resume sleeping, tell yourself, "The next time I'm dreaming, I want to recognize that I'm dreaming." Picture yourself as being back in the dream you've just had; but this time, have your dream-self realize that you are dreaming. Repeat this process until you fall asleep.

You can also follow the lucid-dreaming advice of Don Juan in Carlos Castaneda's *Journey to Ixtlan*: Tell yourself several times before you dream that you are going to look at your hands in your dream, and that this will be a sign to you that you are dreaming. Spend a few moments examining your hands, reminding yourself that you are going to dream of them that night, and then close your eyes and visualize them, repeating your intention.

HYPNOTIC TRANCE

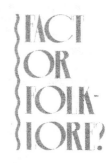

In the popular imagination, the person under hypnosis exhibits a stereotypical look and behavior: glazed or closed eyes, stiff posture, blank facial expression, and an utter absence of initiative—except, of course, when commanded by the hypnotizer to revert to childhood, re-witness a crime, or strut like a rooster. These may not be accurate assessments, but, amazingly, they're the only ones we have. While scientists and laypeople alike have been compelled by experience to admit that hypnosis does exist, so far no one has been able to establish *any* physiological evidence (such as a characteristic brain-wave or heartbeat pattern) for determining whether a person is actually hypnotized.

Is hypnosis a bona fide altered state of consciousness, or is it merely a form of hypersuggestibility? Is it a product of natural brain function, or is it a type of "mental possession" assisted by myths our culture has come to believe?

The modern history of hypnosis has done much to cloud the issue. Historical records of mental states resembling what we know as hypnotic trance go back some three thousand years, but the origin of the present-day name and technique lies in the late eighteenth century, when the Viennese doctor Franz Anton Mesmer created a transatlantic sensation with his new theory of "animal magnetism."

Mesmer believed that the whole universe is permeated by a magnetic fluid and that the stars and the planets cause tides in this fluid that affect the health of human beings. He also believed that human beings are full of magnetic fluid generated by the nerves (a theory close to the "ch'i" theory underlying such Oriental medical practices as acupuncture). Over the years, he extended his theory to include plant life as well. For his cures—and

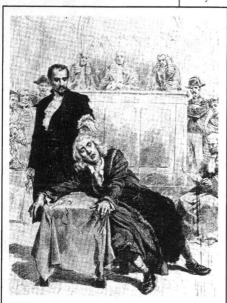

In this nineteenth-century cartoon, Mesmer is shown using hypnotism in a court of law to force a confession from a criminal.

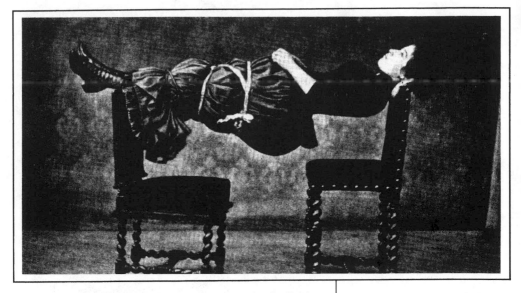

When hypnotists took to the popular stage, one of their most amazing feats was to enable subjects to lie perfectly rigid across the backs of two chairs.

there are many on record—he used iron magnets as well as the magnetism of certain people (like himself) and certain trees to redistribute the sick person's magnetic fluid. The technique came to be called "mesmerism." A pupil of Mesmer's, the Marquis de Puysegur, inadvertently stumbled upon hypnotism while he was trying to mesmerize a young shepherd tied to a magnetic tree. The shepherd fell into a deep trance, and de Puysegur dubbed it "hypnotic" after Hypnos, the Greek god of sleep. Before long, "hypnotism" and "mesmerism" were lumped together in Western languages.

When scientists eventually discredited "mesmerism," they also cast doubt on "hypnotism." Some adventurous researchers continued to experiment with hypnotism as a means of relaxing clients, opening their memories, getting them to speak the truth, or anaesthetizing them from pain. Primarily, however, hypnotism became a conjuring act. In carnivals, circuses, and theaters throughout Europe and America, paid performers with spellbinding voices hypnotized audience members into revealing their weight, lying rigid across two widely spaced chairs, barking like dogs, and letting their fingers be skewered by pins.

Today, because of a renaissance in consciousness studies, hypnotism has gained new respectability. More and more doctors, dentists, psychiatrists, and psychologists are incorporating hypnosis into their practices. Law enforcement professionals are increasingly using hypnosis as a crime-solving tool. And laypeople are hypnotizing themselves in ever greater numbers to break bad habits and reinforce good ones.

The technique of inducing a hypnotic trance is disarmingly simple, but it takes practice to perfect. First, get the subject to remain motionless and yield his or her attention completely to you. Then, encourage drowsiness in the subject by talking him or her into a state of relaxation—the familiar "you are getting sleepy, very sleepy" routine. Adopt a pleasing monotone, varying your language and tone slightly to avoid sounding ridiculous, but not too much. Sometimes it helps to accompany this vocal prompting with a visible item in monotonous motion: a pendulum or one of your fingers moving slowly and surely back and forth in front of the subject's eyes.

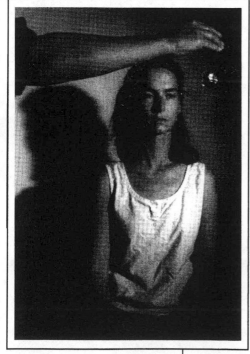

The basics of modern hypnotism are simple and direct: a willing subject and soothing, monotonous inducements to trance.

After a while, you need to make a personal judgment about whether the subject is hypnotized (here's where practice helps). Then you can ask the subject, in a continuously gentle voice, to respond to your requests or suggestions.

The same technique that applies to hypnotizing someone else also applies to self-hypnosis. In the case of self-hypnosis, the vocal inducement is usually silent (mentally "speaking" to yourself) or recorded (listening to your own or someone else's voice on a tape or record). The kinetic visual inducement—if there is one—is something that you don't have to hold, like a metronome or a device that emits soft, regularly-alternating light flashes. The reported benefits of self-hypnosis are legion: People have successfully used it to develop mastery over their emotions and mental energies, to provide assistance in dieting or giving up alcohol or cigarettes, and to overcome phobias like stage fright and fear of flying.

During the hypnotic trance itself, the self-hypnotizer seeks to implant the appropriate "right" attitude and/or behavioral guideline firmly in his or her consciousness. The belief—and often the reality—is that after the trance, it becomes much easier to put this attitude or behavioral guideline into practice. Some advocates claim that self-hypnosis works a bit like self-induced religious conversion: You momentarily experience a wish or desire on a "deeper level" (the so-called "hypnotic suggestion") and, therefore, you are more committed to it in the future.

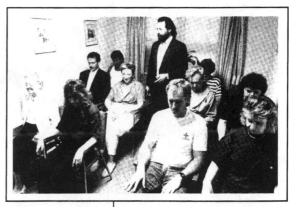

Dr. Martin Sabba, of Clinical Therapy Associates, conducts a Petrie Method stop-smoking seminar that employs hypnotism as a key tool.

While everyone is theoretically capable of being hypnotized, it is true that "highly suggestible" people experience deeper stages of hypnosis. A related trait that favors hypnosis is the ability to "dissociate" easily—to screen information and events from direct conscious awareness. The hypnotic trance experience itself is generally characterized by increased suggestibility, enhanced imagery and imagination (especially pertaining to past memories), lack of will power or decision-making ability, and reality distortions of all kinds (regarding, for example, the passage of time, the naming of objects, the perception of who or what is in the room). In some cases, amnesia relating to the trance can be a natural aftereffect, particularly if the experience has been traumatic. In other cases, amnesia can be an aftereffect if it is suggested during hypnosis. In most cases, however, full memory of the trance is retained.

We may never be able to identify what, exactly, constitutes an hypnotic trance.

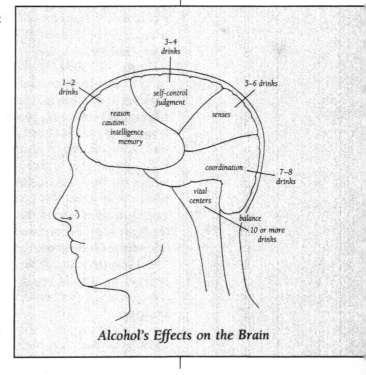

Alcohol's Effects on the Brain

3-4 drinks

1-2 drinks

self-control judgment

5-6 drinks

reason caution intelligence memory

senses

coordination

7-8 drinks

vital centers

balance

10 or more drinks

Neurologists have trouble even guessing what is happening in the brain during hypnosis. In psychological circles, the hypnotic trance is typically classified as a wide range of "discrete" states of consciousness or, more rarely, altered states. Discrete or indiscrete, fact or folklore, hypnosis works, and that may be all we need to know.

Why Can Alcohol Give Me a Hangover, and How Can I Cure It?

Each year, alcohol consumption in the United States is responsible for an estimated 33,000 deaths and $4.5 billion worth of medical expenses, lost income, and decreased productivity, not to mention the incalculable damage it wreaks on the quality of the individual abuser's life and relationships. Fortunately, the vast majority of alcohol consumers do not create or experience any problem worse than an occasional hangover. When that hangover comes, however, it doesn't feel like a minor problem to the sufferer. It can seem as if the entire world is a torture chamber. "Why did I do it?" the anguished victim cries. "How can I stop hurting?"

Usually, the drinker drinks because it feels good. Alcohol is a mild anaesthetic that blocks pain and induces a euphoric state of consciousness. It works on the brain in almost exactly the same, inscrutable way that ether does. If you drink too much, you will fall into a mild coma, just as you will after inhaling a certain quantity of ether. How much alcohol is too much depends on your body weight and rate of metabolism. The average body can metabolize one ounce of 80 proof alcohol (such as a shot of scotch) an hour. Beyond this, you begin to get an increasing disruption of motor faculties as well as more and more perceptual distortion up to mild hallucination.

Lots of factors contribute to making a nightmare out of the morning after. As you drink, the brain eventually compensates for the anaesthetic effect of alcohol by changing its cell walls to become more sensitive. After you stop drinking, you retain this heightened sensitivity for hours or even days. Your head aches, your ears ring, colors are so sharp and vivid they're scary, and any little

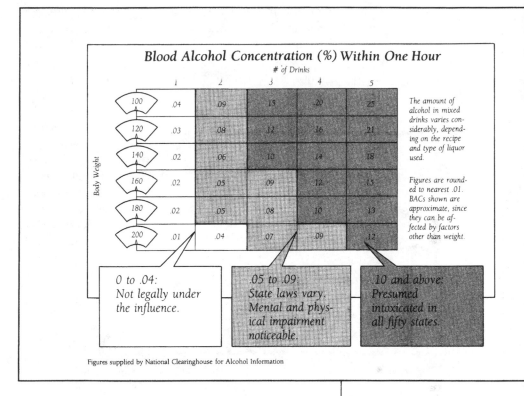

Blood Alcohol Concentration (%) Within One Hour

of Drinks

Body Weight	1	2	3	4	5
100	.04	.09	.15	.20	.25
120	.03	.08	.12	.16	.21
140	.02	.06	.10	.14	.18
160	.02	.05	.09	.12	.15
180	.02	.05	.08	.10	.13
200	.01	.04	.07	.09	.12

The amount of alcohol in mixed drinks varies considerably, depending on the recipe and type of liquor used.

Figures are rounded to nearest .01. BACs shown are approximate, since they can be affected by factors other than weight.

0 to .04:
Not legally under the influence.

.05 to .09:
State laws vary. Mental and physical impairment noticeable.

.10 and above:
Presumed intoxicated in all fifty states.

Figures supplied by National Clearinghouse for Alcohol Information

noise sounds as if it's being amplified tenfold. In addition to this, you're dehydrated, your stomach is queasy, and your motor functions are not kicking in well.

What can you do about it? Aside from making sure not to drink too much or too fast, every drinker has his or her secret. Most of them are best kept secret because they don't work (except, perhaps, psychologically), but here are some suggestions for preventing or treating a hangover that really can be effective:

If the liquor we drank were a pure, laboratory-grade ethyl alcohol, maybe diluted with distilled water, we'd be a lot better off. Most of what we drink is impure—full of yeast or sugar (for fermentation) and/or flavoring and coloring agents. As a result, disruptive chemicals known as congeners are left in our brain and body to add to our troubles. In terms of alcohol purity, it's wiser to drink vodka rather than bourbon, white wine than red wine. It can make a big difference in how you feel the next day.

- Fatty, oily food eaten before drinking helps to line the stomach and delay or impede drunkenness. To a lesser degree, a glass of milk also functions this way. Drinking on an empty stomach (no food for three hours) definitely assists drunkenness.

A scientific definition of a poet might put it something like this: A man of an extraordinarily sensitive and active subconscious personality, fed by, and feeding, a nonresistant consciousness.
—Amy Lowell

- Eating cabbage the next day can help rid your system of congeners, since cabbage is an ideal chelator, or absorber of congeners. Russian drinkers often turn to borscht the next day; Germans, to sauerkraut. It's also a good idea to consume fructose (as in honey) the day after drinking: It helps to bolster your metabolism, and, therefore, the alcohol in your system will burn off more quickly. Since alcohol kills vitamins, you may want to take a vitamin supplement. Unfortunately, hot coffee, the traditional cure for drunkenness as well as hangovers, is of no avail in either case—although it may act as a placebo, thanks to widespread popular belief in its powers.

- Any exercise after (or during) drinking works to increase your metabolism and hurry alcohol through your system. Rolling naked in the snow is ideal, since it gets your blood pumping particularly fast, but so are more pleasurable activities like walking, dancing, or making love. The more sedentary drinker can take a sauna bath and accomplish the same thing (although you risk passing out if you take a sauna bath *while* you are drinking).

- The famous "hair-of-the-dog" cure has a sound scientific basis. A modest amount of alcohol the next day acts as a buffer for your hypersensitive brain cells and allows them to return gradually to their normal state. Many drinkers swear by bitters the next morning (specifically,

Fernet Branca), a glass of beer, or a Bloody Mary. There's even a Hair of the Dog cocktail that includes beneficial fructose: Take one and a half ounces of scotch and add one tablespoon of honey and one tablespoon of double cream. Shake it with ice, strain, and serve. Limit yourself to one, however, or you may end up back where you started.

Do Subliminal Messages Really Work?

As the legend goes, it happened at a New Jersey drive-in movie theater in 1956, during a screening of the movie *Picnic*. Without the audience's knowledge, an invisible message flashed across the screen every thirty-two seconds: "Eat popcorn. Drink Coke." Lo and behold, the theater concession stand was besieged all evening by hungry and thirsty patrons.

Marketers still spin this yarn, and psychologists still try to unravel its meaning. Dr. Howard Shevrin of the University of Michigan, who has made a thirty-year study of subliminal perception and "unconscious" learning, feels that it can't work so predictably, especially if the message itself doesn't address some issue that is already important to the receiver. "A subject given a subliminal message relating to an internal conflict he's having does respond with unique, measurable brain patterns," Shevrin points out, "but he can respond in many different ways. Some messages may exacerbate a conflict rather than solve it."

Suppose, for example, that you are using audio tapes to feed the subliminal message "I love my father" to a young man who resents the dominating influence his father has on his life. The young man's response may be to feel more love for his father and, correspondingly, less resentment. Or the young man may feel more frustrated about his resentment, which remains just as strong but is now being accompanied by sensations of love. Or the young man may develop even more resentment toward his father because he is unable to feel the love he is "inexplicably" being directed to feel. It's a somewhat crude example, but it illustrates the opinion of many psychologists that subliminal messages have no guarantee of producing specific results.

Such pronouncements have had little adverse effect on the booming market for self-help audio cassette tapes containing subliminal messages. The promises are irresistible: Without putting out any "conscious" effort, you can strengthen your will power, improve your memory, sharpen your golf game, overcome stuttering, stop the spread of disease in your body, and radiate more sexual confidence. Most tapes feature a subaudible message (motivational, instructional, and/or incantory) recorded beneath a pleasingly neutral audible track, such as the sound of ocean waves. Some tapes include an audible version of the message on a second side, while others overlay the subliminal message with an audible track that can be used for self-hypnotic suggestion.

The center

that I cannot find
is known to my unconscious mind.
—W. H. Auden

Despite the fact that academics scoff at the tapes, most users claim significant results, and so subliminal messages are rapidly attracting new adherents and new applications. Students are experimenting with learning in their sleep through tapes. Parents are playing educational and confidence-building messages in the nursery. Free from any legal restraints on the matter, managers are using subliminal suggestion to create a happy workforce, to discourage theft in stores, to promote gambling in casinos, and to deter rowdiness in public assembly areas. In the fall of 1988, Dallas radio station KMEZ-FM broadcast twelve-minute stop-smoking subliminal messages at preannounced times. Ken Loomis, program director, reports, "The voice behind the music was reasoning with you, suggesting why you should quit. The switchboard went crazy with people who were enthusiastic about the idea."

The jury is definitely out on the potential effectiveness of subliminal messages in visual formats. Several years ago, a major distiller ran an enormously successful magazine ad featuring a close-up of a glass of whiskey on the rocks. Some amateur critics claimed that erotic images were cleverly concealed in the melting patterns of the ice cubes, causing the viewer to make a subconscious connection between the product and sex. The distiller acknowledged that a viewer might see provocative shapes in the cubes but denied that these shapes were intentionally put there. Whether or not such a connection did—or could—spur sales is impossible to prove. There's also no hard-core evidence that a person in a coma can subconsciously attend to the spoken or broadcast word, although there's a large body of anecdotal material suggesting that it may happen.

Meanwhile, back at the movie theater, operators assure us that we are not going to be subjected to anything like the alleged 1956 *Picnic* invasion of the subconscious snatchers. But, then, how would we know if we were?

◆◆◆◆◆◆◆◆◆◆

A dream which is

not understood is like a letter which is not opened.
—Talmud

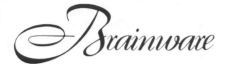

Brainware

Isolation Tank

The granddaddy of all contemporary devices meant to induce altered states of consciousness, the isolation tank has become more or less standard equipment in university research labs, mental health facilities, and personal growth centers across the United States. Users typically spend ten minutes to a half hour floating on their back in a soundproof, lightproof tank filled with ten inches of water that contains up to 800 pounds of Epsom salts—enough to keep the body perfectly buoyant, with the ears underwater. The water temperature is so close to that of the body that there's no feeling of separation between the skin and the water. Brain waves assume slower and deeper patterns, and the mind, free of virtually all physical sensations (except, perhaps, for the sounds of internal organs) is thereby inclined to produce the types of hallucinatory and potentially illuminating impressions that are associated with dreams and drug trips. For aquaphobes who prefer dry isolation, there's a box called Superspace that employs a very floppy waterbed with a velvetized skin to achieve similar results.

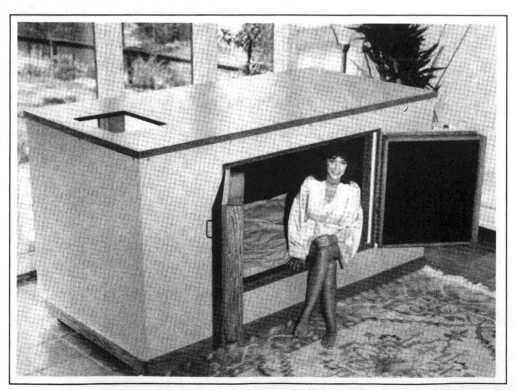

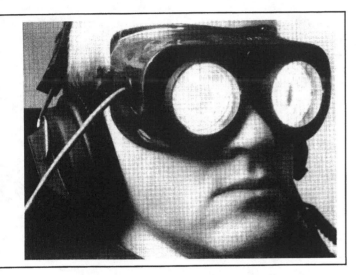

Synchro-Energizer

The Synchro-Energizer is now being hailed by many New Age self-helpers as the Nautilus machine of the mind. Currently the star attraction at brain spas in major American cities, the head-borne apparatus combines flickering lights, pulsating sounds, and vibrating electromagnetic impulses to influence brain-wave activity. It doesn't matter, advocates claim, how that activity is altered; as long as it differs from "normal" activity, it will refresh and retool one's state of consciousness. In many cases, the user also lies suspended in a large padded disk, to increase his or her detachment from hard reality. According to the machine's creator, Denis E. Gorges, the benefits of synchro-energizing for twenty minutes can result in up to a week of "deep internal relaxation" or even "more harmonic cooperation between the right brain and the left brain." For interested parties who do not live within driving distance of a brain spa, there are portable models to use at home. Resembling a portable stereo connected to a pair of headphone/goggles, the typical mechanism features an entire sound-and-light program prerecorded on a cassette.

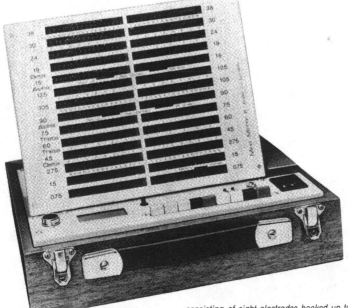

Mind Mirror

The Mind Mirror, lately gaining popularity as a corporate training instrument in addition to being a brain spa favorite, was eight years in the making. First, the inventors wired up Indian yogi volunteers to determine the electroencephalogram (EEG) pattern produced by an "awakened mind," which is essentially a Theta pattern of brain waves. Then they devised a machine consisting of eight electrodes hooked up to a gridlike screen on which the user can see his or her own EEG pattern. Through a combination of forming euphoric mental images, breathing rhythmically, monitoring his or her EEG pattern for biofeedback, and comparing that pattern to the "awakened mind" pattern, the user can learn to achieve something akin to the "feeling tone" of an advanced yogi. Whether or not individual users realize this particular goal, they can almost certainly come to recognize and appreciate what the Alpha brain-wave level (a relaxed, meditative state) feels like and how best to go about engendering it.

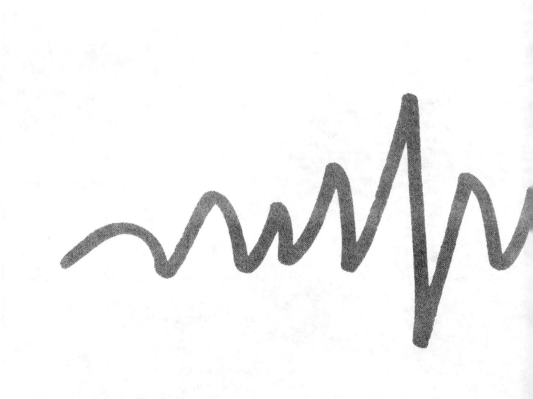

3
MEMORY

*I*n ancient Greek mythology, Mnemosyne (memory) gives birth to the nine muses: Clio (history), Urania (astronomy and sacred mysteries), Melpomene (tragedy), Thalia (comedy), Terpsichore (dance), Calliope (epic poetry), Erato (love poetry), Polyhymnia (religious poetry), and Euterpe (lyric poetry and music). Thus the ancient Greeks acknowledged the importance of memory to the creative arts—those modes of expression that testify most persuasively to the divine spirit in human beings. In fact, memory is the vital source of *all* aspects of human intelligence, imagination, and accomplishment. We could not reason, daydream, or tie our shoes, much less compose grand opera, were it not for our brain's power to record and recall past experience.

Pervasive function that it is, memory resists any easy definition. Take the simple act of remembering a face. There's a big difference between *recognizing* that face and *recalling* that face. Our memory of a specific face when we see it may go no further than the recognition level: We are aware that we've encountered it before, yet we can't attach a name to it, and, chances are, we haven't mentally envisioned that face since we last came across it. But if we recall the face when we see it, that means we are able to give it a name and, therefore, we are more likely to have thought about it during the time since we last saw it.

We can also define memories differently on the basis of duration. *Short-term memory* refers to the ability of the brain to pick up and retain new information automatically for a few seconds or perhaps as long as several hours if we pay particular attention to it. Afterward we forget it altogether. This is the common fate of grocery lists, little-used phone numbers, and the sequence of events in the course of an unremarkable day. These bits and pieces may be stored in our memory system along with every other detail in our life experience, but if they are, we quickly lose the ability to retrieve them. *Long-term memories,* by contrast, can last a lifetime. We may be able to retrieve them whenever we choose, or they may only come back to us under certain favorable circumstances. Whether or not a given fact or impression crosses the boundary between short-term memory and long-term memory depends on how frequently our mind returns to it during the day it first comes to us and during the days, weeks, months, and even years that follow.

Finally, the memory process varies according to the na-

<figure>
outside stimuli

Impressions not attended to

rehearsal

sight
hearing
touch
taste
smell

short-term memory → elaborative process → long-term memory

retrieval

decay → permanently lost

forgetting → permanently lost

forgetting → lost or unavailable but possibly recoverable
</figure>

ture of what we're remembering. *Episodic memory* involves the retention of interrelated times, places, and circumstances, while *semantic memory* involves the retention of individual facts and ideas. Amnesiacs, for instance, may lose track of whole chapters in their past (episodic memories) and yet still hold on to all their academic and professional knowledge (semantic memories). They may forget their name because it is tied to their ongoing personal history, but they may not forget the names of the planets, which they originally set about remembering in a more detached, disciplined way. Then there are *skill memories*. These are the task-performance memories we acquire by practice that eventually turn into virtual habits. We rely on such memories to drive a car, play the piano, swim the breaststroke, and button our coats. Skill memory is the most primitive form of memory and the least likely to be touched by amnesia or any other memory disorder.

> ## "I did that,"
> says my memory. "I could not have done that," says my pride, and remains inexorable. Eventually, the memory yields, hiding till the desire for truth overcomes my pride.
>
> —Friedrich Nietzsche

Picturing how the memory works is even more complicated than defining the different kinds of memory. Scientists used to think that the brain's memory was organized like a library—each bit of data "shelved" in its own cell and recalled by stimulation of that cell. Now we know that the memory's storage-and-retrieval system is far more sophisticated. The brain does not file images as they are received. Instead, new information is transformed into a flow-stream pattern of electrochemical transmissions among a series of cells, a pattern that serves to incorporate that information into an intricate network of preexisting knowledge. In this way, the memory of a specific red brick house becomes intermeshed with every memory featuring redness, bricks, and houses, as well as with associative memories having to do with the house's location, size, history, and so forth. Presumably, different memories share portions of the same neural circuits. Most definitely, each of our individual memories winds up being connected with, and influenced by, all our other memories.

Given how our memory is organized and how our memory operates, it is not surprising that our ability to remember something well rests on three principles: repetition, interest, and association. Repetition is self-explanatory; the more we reiterate a fact or impression, the deeper we ingrain it into our memory system. The interest principle works more subtly. If we're already fascinated by a particular subject—be it geology, football, Ireland, or movie stars—then we're naturally more likely to retain new details linked to it. After all, the parts of our consolidated memory network relating to that body of knowledge are much more richly articulated and much more frequently accessed in our day-to-day lives than other parts. If, however, we lack a natural interest in certain bits of new information, we can still command ourselves to take an interest. Through sheer willful concentration when we first learn them, we can increase the potential that we'll remember the names of people we meet at a party or the theorems we study in a math book.

Not all decisions regarding interest, however, lie within our power to make. The culture in which we live conditions us to be more interested in some types of information than others. Australian psychologist Judith Kearins found that Aborigine children perform markedly better than children of European stock in exercises that require remembering the size, shape, and arrangement of stones. The reason, she contends, is that the Aborigine culture places more value on establishing one's relationship with the physical environment. In a study conducted by a British researcher, Liberian farmers tested worse than their urban counterparts at recalling new wordlists (such as "sun, coat, three, road, purple, dog"), but better at recalling new stories. The two tasks require roughly the same kind of memory skill, but the culture of the farmer favors

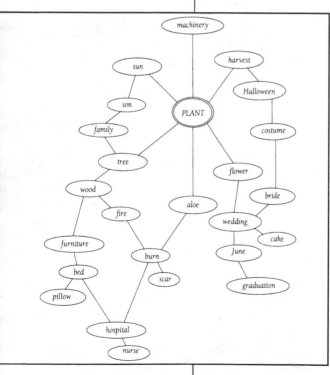

The brain differs significantly from a computer in its ability to interrelate a wide range of images through a process of creative association, as suggested by this semantic network.

narrative communication—the recounting of events and situations—whereas the culture of the city-dweller favors data communication—the recitation of facts and figures.

The most effective memory-building techniques of all are based on the principle of association. The more connections we deliberately create between new information and information that is already familiar to us, the better our brain can retain that new information and recall it at a later date. Suppose you want to remember some financial advice you've just read in a waiting-room magazine article. If you take the time to visualize yourself following that advice and to think about how it compares to other alternatives, you will consolidate it more firmly in your memory system. You can also increase the likelihood that you'll remember it if you make the effort to associate that article with the setting in which you've just read it. Associative memory aids can even be fictitious. Assuming you want to remember a list of complicated medical terms, it helps to fabricate a distinctive mental picture for each term, or to substitute a more memorable sound-alike word or phrase for each term, or to imagine each term attached to a road sign in a well-known street map.

This chapter will assist you to understand and enhance your brain's memory capabilities. It surveys each level of memory proficiency—from amnesia, to simple forgetful-

The Nose Knows

Whatever the evolutionary logic, our senses of smell and taste (taste being a dependent relative of our sense of smell) are uniquely positioned to create and evoke memories. The explanation requires a close look at how the brain remembers. The absorption of data into the brain's memory system is technically termed "consolidation." The consolidated memory system is located in the cerebral cortex—the largest and most developed portion of the human brain. And the agent that mysteriously routes first-time information into the consolidated memory system is the tiny hippocampus in the center of the brain, right next door to the locus for registering smell and taste (the only senses not initially processed via the lower brain and cortex).

As it turns out, smell and taste are singularly strong memory triggers. The perfume industry capitalizes on the powerful proximity of the smell and taste receptors to the hippocampus ("Her Windsong stays on my mind . . ."). So does the food industry, which emphasizes the nostalgia value of all sorts of products from homemade-style soups to oven-fresh chocolate chip cookies. And so do the arts. The French novelist Marcel Proust attributes the inspiration for his masterpiece Remembrance of Things Past to the aroma and taste of a madeleine tea cake, which instantly carries him back to his boyhood in Cambray. The implication seems to be that if you yearn to take a sentimental journey, follow your nose!

ness, to photographic memory—and draws lessons from it that can help you help yourself to a better memory. You will also receive guidance on living a more memorable life, through appreciating how your age and your brain's moment-to-moment state of being affects the way your memory works. In addition, you will gain insights into some of the core mysteries associated with memory, including major theories about what causes déjà vu, possible explanations for past-life recall, and the manner in which diets and drugs may actually improve or rehabilitate your brain's memory system.

Why Do I Forget Things, and What Can I Do About It?

When we forget who loaned us a book, where we parked the car, whether we've taken our vitamins yet, or even why we've just walked into the kitchen, it's an invitation to panic. Are we getting senile? Is brain damage from years of jug wine and potato chips finally kicking in? Is our present life-style so mentally unstimulating that our mind is turning to mush?

Generally speaking, the answer to each of these questions is no. Simple forgetfulness is common regardless of one's age, diet, or way of life. It's even healthy. Individual memory impressions can be too strong for our own good, generating all sorts of fears, phobias, obsessions, and preoccupations. And if we remembered everything perfectly, we might share the fate of Jorge Luis Borges's short story character Irineo Funes ("Funes the Memory Man"), whose inability to lose track of details drives him insane.

Dr. Ulric Neisser of Emory University and Dr. Douglas Herrman of Hamilton College recently surveyed over 200 people to determine which types of simple memory lapses happen most frequently. At the top of the list were: forgetting the name of someone a few minutes after being introduced; being unable to remember any details of a dream after awakening with the strong sense of having dreamed; and forgetting to bring up a point in a conversation. Further down on the list were such items as going out and leaving something behind and not remembering the exact date.

Granted that it is common to forget things, what are the usual causes of such forgetfulness? It could be that the sequential pattern of brain-cell stimulation necessary to make the memory connection is temporarily out-of-whack. Maybe part of that pattern is being used for some other purpose at the moment, for example, thinking about an appointment, and the result is a kind of "crossing of the lines"; or maybe at one stage of the process there's a fraction-of-a-second delay or speeding up that throws the rest of the process off track.

Often the problem is one of perception, not memory. We've all had the maddening experience of being unable to find our keys after rummaging far and wide, only to have someone else find them for us where we first

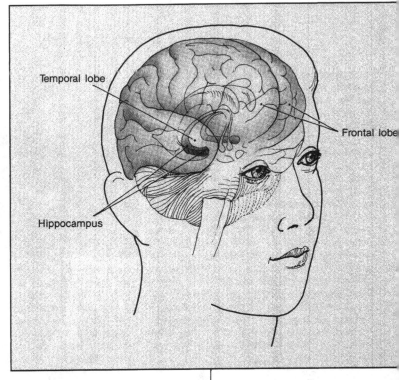

Temporal lobe

Frontal lobe

Hippocampus

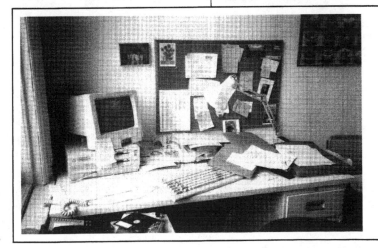

Neatness is not always in the memory's best interest. Consider the office space pictured here. Individual papers on the desk, the bulletin board, and even the lamp may be easier for their user to locate precisely because they are left in offbeat, personally significant places and positions.

Walking Encyclopedias

In a remote forest in Europe, dropouts from a repressive, book-burning regime wander among the birches, repeating to themselves banned literary masterpieces that they've memorized. It's a haunting image in Ray Bradbury's futuristic novel Fahrenheit 451, especially for anyone who was ever challenged in school to memorize a whole poem, speech, or story word for word.

On the whole, our formal education discourages such memorization and trains us to rely instead on a wide range of external memory aids, such as notes, outlines, tapes, and reference books. These aids greatly expand the amount of "recallable" data we have at our disposal, but they also encourage us to become lazy-brained. We don't keep adequate mental records of our daily schedules or errand lists because we have them written down. We don't bother remembering what we're reading because we know we possess a permanent text. We put off thinking about important projects until we're sitting at our desks, surrounded by such reassuring and seemingly all-important memory props as paper and pencil, folder and file, hardware and software.

From the time of the muse-worshipping Greeks until shortly after the invention of the printing press, people placed high value on memorization; and predigious feats of memory were commonplace. Otherwise, entire

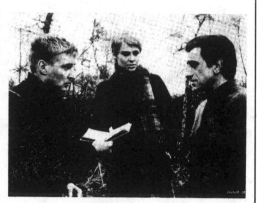

epics, histories, genealogies, religious philosophies, and scientific protocols would have been lost to the ages. In the post-printing-press era, human memory powers have been sadly undervalued and neglected. The famous American psychologist William James, concerned in the early 1900s about whether he was capable of meeting the type of memory challenge that many people met prior to the 1500s, set himself the task of memorizing all of John Milton's twelve-book poetic saga Paradise Lost. It took him a month; and the result was, in his words, "supremely inspirational."

Oskar Werner (left) and Julie Christie starred in François Truffaut's film version of Ray Bradbury's novel Fahrenheit 451. Oskar Werner was, in fact, a refugee from Nazi Germany, where real book burnings were conducted.

searched. However familiar an object may be, if it doesn't look quite the way we expect it to look, we may *see* it without *recognizing* it. Alternatively, we may not want to recognize the object we're seeking. Assuming we must start working on an onerous task once we find the object, we may harbor a subliminal desire never to see it again. This desire can keep us from concentrating during the hunt. Forgetting whos, whats, whys, and whens may result from similar perceptual difficulties. Somehow we can't connect, or don't want to connect, the "missing" information with our state of mind at the moment.

Problems contributing to memory lapses can also be organizational in nature. The well-meaning person who straightens up our messy desk may, in fact, be doing us a big disservice. What appears to be chaos to that person may actually be an arrangement uniquely calculated to fit our memory needs. "We structure our surroundings, in large part, so that they act as a memory aid," says Donald Norman, a cognitive psychologist at the University of California at San Diego. "People make a sort of natural map of their world by putting things in places that fit their habits. When there is no fit between where things are and what you need them for, then memory is more likely to fail." [Quoted from "Forgetfulness Is Seen Causing More Worry Than It Should" by Daniel Goleman, *New York Times,* July 1, 1986.]

In a like manner, we may forget pieces of information because they are not situated well in our overall memory's frame of reference. We can't recall who loaned us a book because we lack a good mental "filing cue" linking that particular book with its owner: for example, an association of the cover design with the owner's "style," or a memory of a conversation with the owner about the subject of the book. We can't remember why we've come into the kitchen because it was an impulsive decision—one that we responded to without thinking and, therefore, without connecting it well to the physical and mental events surrounding it.

How, then, can we cope with our less than perfect memories and make sure that they are as effective as they need to be? The basic steps are as follows:

Spend Time Remembering. Before performing any of your daily activities—running errands, making a presentation at work, dining with friends—take a few minutes to go over all the things you want to remember. Don't rely on notes to do all the memory work for you. Rehearse in your mind what you want to say to others. Visualize yourself doing what you want to do.

When circumstances present you with something you'd like to remember—a person's name, the location of a store, a great idea—give yourself a moment or two right away to repeat and absorb the new information. Try associating it with other facts and images so that you have more memory hooks for retrieving it later.

After an event, conduct a personal "mental review" of

what took place, focusing tightly on details that you believe are worth retaining.

During your leisure time in general, pursue activities that will exercise your powers of memory, such as doing crossword puzzles, learning stories to tell a child, or reviewing old scrapbooks.

Buy Time When You've Forgotten. If you typically need more time to recall things on demand, build this time into your response. Smile or clear your throat to give yourself a few seconds to cover a memory lapse in a conversation. When you're stuck in a rut trying to remember a specific detail, stop trying and start doing something altogether different: The desired detail is apt to pop into your mind later, when you're not straining so hard to remember it. Rather than waste time or make errors when you can't remember a whole body of information in the course of a business meeting, set up a later time to get back to it.

Organize Your Life So That It Is More Memorable. At night, make to-do lists for the next day. Create special resting spots for objects that you're inclined to misplace: a peg on which to hang your keys when you enter your home or a box in which to drop each bill as it arrives. Schedule recurring activities so that you always handle them at the same time of the day, week, or month. It might sound monotonous, but it could be your salvation!

Have Confidence in Your Memory. Our memory lives up to what we expect of it, and most of us underrate our memory. Consequently, we're apt to be anxiety-ridden when we know we have to remember something. Anxiety, alas, is a surefire forgetting mechanism. Worse, we may not even make the effort to remember something, being so convinced that we won't be able to remember it. Work on having a good attitude about your memory. Stop blaming your innate powers of memory—which are staggering—and start telling yourself that it's up to you to help your powers of memory work. Relax prior to facing any situation that will challenge your memory, such as a test, a social gathering, or a business meeting. Give your memory time and attention, and it will serve you well.

AMNESIACS

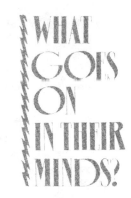

WHAT GOES ON IN THEIR MINDS?

On November 17, 1912, one of the most farfetched and yet popular plot devices in fiction occurred in the real life of a famous writer. Sherwood Anderson, the author of *Winesburg, Ohio,* was sitting in his Elyria, Ohio, office dictating a letter to his secretary. Suddenly he stopped in mid-sentence and strode out of the room. He wasn't seen again until four days later, when he was spotted in a Cleveland drugstore, dazed and disoriented, and rushed to Hudson Road Hospital. Doctors there determined that he was the victim of amnesia caused by mental strain. For the rest of his life, he spun stories of those missing days for his family and friends, each time with different details. He simply could not recall what actually happened.

Almost any severe strain, injury, or disease of the brain can cause loss of memory without damaging other mental functions. In most cases, however, pure amnesia—the absence of a significant time-block of memories—results from a blow to the head, a stroke, or oxygen deprivation in the brain due to a blood clot or an overdose of anaesthesia.

The most common form of amnesia is called *antero-grade*: The victim can't recall anything that happens after the onset of memory loss for longer than an hour. Usually the victim resumes having longer memories within days, weeks, or months of the loss episode, but he or she may remain stuck in the past forever, constantly believing that "now" is the time period just before the memory loss happened and that he or she has not grown any older.

This latter dilemma almost always befalls people who suffer from Korsakov's syndrome, brought on by excessive alcohol consumption over many years, coupled with a poor diet that robs the brain of thiamine, a vitamin necessary for good memory function. When confronted by the fact that time has, indeed, marched on (for example, by being forced to study their face in a mirror or current events in a newspaper), Korsakov victims panic and fumble for their sanity until a few moments go by and they forget that they've forgotten. Ironically their history of subterfuge and make believe as alcoholics can often prove a life-saver in one respect—they somehow manage to survive by concealing their handicap from themselves as well as others.

Far less common—except in romance novels, television detective shows, and soap operas—is *retrograde amnesia,* in which the victim can only remember what's happened since losing his or her memory, or *global amnesia,* in which the loss of memory is virtually total and recovery is much less likely. "Clive," an English musicologist, organist, and choral master, developed global amnesia after suffering an attack of encephalitis that destroyed his brain's hippocampus (an important memory-processing center in the limbic system). Now Clive lives in an eternal present. He knows who he is and can recognize his wife, but his consciousness is reduced to a span of moments.

Confined for safety and observation purposes to a hospital room, Clive keeps a diary. Each entry is sadly the same: "Now I am completely awake, for the first time in years." If he is directed to look back in his diary, he claims not to remember writing the previous entries and denies that he is the author. Whenever his wife enters the room, even if she's only been gone for a few minutes, he greets her ecstatically as if he's been separated from her for years.

"He sees what is right in front of him," Clive's wife explains, "but as soon as that information hits the brain, it fades. Nothing makes an impression, nothing registers. Everything goes in perfectly well, because he has all his faculties. His intellect is virtually intact, and he perceives the world as you or I do. But as soon as he perceives it and looks away, it's gone for him."

Not all global amnesiacs are helpless. A Michigan woman was overcome by global amnesia after an aneurysm operation several years ago; but, relying on her intact IQ of 145 and her ability to recall events as far back as fifteen minutes, she follows a detailed written schedule to conduct an independent and fulfilling life. She checks off each preplanned event as it happens, so she'll know she's done it. When she goes on vacation, she write numerous postcards to herself every day so she can "recollect" the trip when she's back home. "Most people's lives are an accumulation of the past," she says. "Mine no longer is. I decided to optimize the present."

What Is a Photographic Memory, and Can I Develop One?

If we're not one of them, we learn to know them and hate them in grade school—the kids who can look once at a map of state capitals, or a table of elements, or a list of commonly misspelled words and hours later recall everything they've seen, down to finger smudges and mustard stains in the margins. These individuals are blessed with what we've come to call in the twentieth century a "photographic memory" (technically speaking, a "visual-image memory"). Somehow, their brains can almost effortlessly retain information in its originally perceived format.

No doubt about it, a photographic memory greatly assists any intellectual or creative endeavor. The famous American conductor Arturo Toscanini, for example, used his photographic memory to keep a mental record of every note for every instrument in 100 operas and 250 symphonies. It wasn't an "all-purpose talent," he insisted—he had to have a strong incentive to remember the material he studied. Unfortunately for would-be imitators, however, his remarkable skill *was* an innate talent. We can train ourselves to remember things more efficiently and effectively, but we have to be born with a photographic memory.

By most estimates, only one out of ten children enters the world with a photographic memory, and nine of those ten lucky children lose their special ability by the time they're adults. Therefore, a mere 1 percent of the adult population is gifted with photographic memory. When the other 99 percent look at a picture and close their eyes, they retain a precisely duplicate after-image (called an "iconic" memory) for one-tenth of a second and a reasonably duplicate after-image for up to a couple of seconds. When people with photographic memories look at a picture, they retain both types of after-images for much longer time periods.

Researchers once asked a woman who was reputed to have a photographic memory to look with her left eye through the red lens of a pair of glasses similar to 3-D goggles. She saw 10,000 red dots that the lens made visible on a sheet of paper. Then she looked through the neighboring green lens with her right eye and saw a different set of 10,000 green dots. When the researchers asked her to describe the complicated image that would result from combining both sets of dots, she was able to do so immediately, thanks to her perfect recall of each set.

While we may never become this adept, we can strengthen our visual memory through repeated practice. Every so often, take a few minutes and try this experiment.

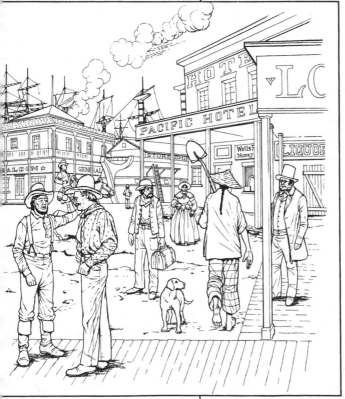

Using this picture, try the experiment outlined in the text for strengthening your visual memory.

• Hold your head straight and examine the scene in front of you: whether it is a picture, a room, or an outdoor setting. First, move your eyes slowly from right to left and back again, keeping track of what you see. Then, move your eyes down from the top and back up again, keeping track of what you see.

• After about thirty seconds, close your eyes. Recall as clearly as you can what objects exist in that scene: from right to left, from left to right, from top to bottom, and from bottom to top.

• Open your eyes and see how successful you were. What objects did you remember well? Remember poorly? Forget? Recall in the wrong order? What objects now look somehow different or less impressive or more impressive than when you first examined them?

• Repeat the experiment and, afterward, compare your two performances.

Are There Drugs or Medicines That Can Improve My Memory?

Begone, tedious drills, expensive therapy, and spooky hypnosis! Isn't there some substance we can swallow or inject into our bloodstream that will increase our powers of memory or at least repair memory damage caused by injury or disease?

Down through the ages, human beings have searched diligently for just such a substance. Today, anthropologists report, natives of Borneo living with Stone Age technology are still eating the brains of dead relatives, friends, and enemies in an effort to absorb their memory banks. Meanwhile, their Western World contemporaries are just beginning to investigate the possibility of a memory drug with a more fastidious chemical or hormonal base.

At the University of Toronto, nutritionist Carol Leprohon-Greenwood has discovered that rats fed with soybean oil are 15 percent better at performing memory experiments than rats fed with lard. This doesn't necessarily mean we should be consuming large quantities of soybean oil to sharpen our memories, but it does suggest that replacing saturated fats in our diet with polyunsaturated fats could help. The fatty membranes of the neurons responsible for memory function in the brain are known to harden with age, and polyunsaturated fats keep them pliant and more efficient at carrying electrochemical signals.

Rats have also assisted humans in discovering another potential memory drug: an experimental compound called vinpocetine, now under development at Ayerst Laboratories in New York City. Vinpocetine works as a catalyst to make neurons use glucose more effectively—a major factor in the memory-transmission process. Assuming vinpocetine passes all its tests, though, it won't do much good for healthy people who are simply forgetful by nature. The principal beneficiaries will be people whose memory has been physically impaired by a stroke.

Enhancing "normal" memory systems poses a much more complicated challenge than restoring damaged

Photographic Evidence

On the left is a PET scan of a normal brain. On the right is a PET scan of the brain of a sixty-five-year-old housewife suffering from Alzheimer's disease. Her particular loss of memory function has resulted in an inability to perform such everyday visual–spatial tasks as dressing herself, making her bed, and setting the table. This shows up in the PET scan as a severe impairment to the right side of her brain. (See Chapter 1 for more information on PET scans and right brain/left brain functions.)

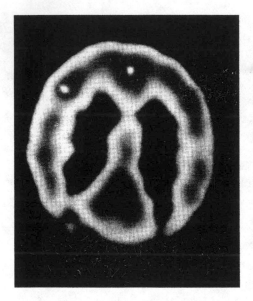 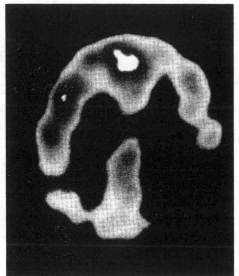

memory systems. Because our memories work better when we're alert, aroused, and/or motivated, researchers have long assumed that the energy-boosting hormone adrenaline might be used as a normal memory stimulant. Enter, once again, the hard-working rat. James McGaugh of the University of California at Irvine has convincingly demonstrated that rats injected with adrenaline do, indeed, remember far longer.

In the laboratory of human experience, evidence abounds to support McGaugh's findings. For example, most people who were teenage or older when President John F. Kennedy was assassinated in 1963 can still remember precise details of where they were, what they were doing, and how they felt that day. The shocking news sent adrenaline rushing through their brain, and, as a result, their memory impressions associated with that news are more indelible and easier to recall than typical-day memories. Adrenaline, however, is a very strong hormone with far-reaching effects throughout the body. So—rats!—we don't yet have a safe, memory-specific application for adrenaline. But science is still working on it.

A more promising line of research has to do with a neurotransmitter called acetylcholine. This chemical seems to be important in memory-processing and is significantly deficient in many cases in Alzheimer's disease, which ranks as the most common cause of memory loss. Many doctors are now treating their Alzheimer patients with acetylcholine-boosting drugs, usually containing some form of lecithin.

In one doctor's study, some Alzheimer patients showed significant memory improvement after several months of drinking two milkshakes daily, each containing 35 grams of 53 percent phosphatidylcholine-content lecithin granules. Another study conducted by Dr. Richard Levy of the Maudsley Hospital in London resulted in half of his Alzheimer patients exhibiting better memory ability after receiving large, regular doses of lecithin over a six-month period.

To date, such treatment for Alzheimer patients can only postpone the death of the brain cells that manufacture acetylcholine; it can't prevent those cells from dying or replace their function once they do die. Treated patients' memories perform better for a while than the memories of nontreated patients, but both groups are condemned, eventually, to the same degree of memory loss.

While science continues exploring ways to prevent the death of acetylcholine-producing cells in Alzheimer patients, thousands of diet-conscious people are responding to the available research by taking lecithin supplements to keep their normal memory systems in top shape. Soon they can turn to a legendary source of good health—chicken soup. In the near future, Thomas J. Lipton, Inc. plans to market a new product consisting of its basic chicken noodle soup laced with lecithin. Although regulatory restrictions prevent Lipton from labeling this concoction "Memory Soup," it's about as close to it as we can get!

STATE-BOUND KNOWLEDGE

WORDS FOR THE WISE

In Charlie Chaplin's classic film *City Lights,* Charlie the Tramp prevents a drunken millionaire from committing suicide. In gratitude, the millionaire embraces Charlie and invites him to move into his mansion. The next morning, the sober millionaire has no memory of the incident and kicks Charlie out. And so it goes throughout the film. Whenever he's drunk, the millionaire fawns on Charlie as if he were his long-lost best friend, but as soon as the millionaire sobers up, he forgets the connection altogether.

Roland Fischer, a frequent contributor to *Psychology Today* magazine, cites this plot to illustrate what scientists have termed "state-bound knowledge." The theory behind state-bound knowledge is that the brain processes and stores information differently at each separate level of consciousness: sober or drunk, alert or tired, excited or calm, happy or sad. As a result, each bit of information we acquire winds up being attached to, and most easily remembered at, one particular conscious state. "The greater the difference between these states," Fischer says, "the more difficult it is to recall in one state specifics learned in another." Gordon Bower, a psychologist at Stanford University, puts it this way: "It is as though the two states constitute different libraries into which a person places memory records. A given memory record can be retrieved only by returning to that library, or physiological state, in which the event was first stored." (See Chapter 2, "Consciousness," for tips on remembering images from your dreams.)

Seldom is the rift between memory and forgetfulness so complete as it is for Charlie's millionaire, or for others who suffer alcoholic blackouts, or for mind-explorers who are unable to recapture back on Earth the otherworldly wonders they've encountered under the influence of drugs or mystic ecstasy. Nevertheless, the existence of state-bound knowledge may explain why so many of us have trouble remembering incidents from our childhood—we're incapable of accessing the states of mind we experienced then. Perhaps the psychiatrist's couch works so well to put us more in touch with our earliest years because it relaxes us so quickly and completely, producing slower brain-wave rhythms, which are similar to those in which young children spend a considerable amount of their time.

Certainly we're all familiar with how effectively old songs evoke buried memories of old loves. The mood stirred up by the lyrics and music refreshes our connection with past episodes colored by the same mood. Most of us also go through the bittersweet experience of formulating great plans or ideas while we're on vacation, only to lose complete track of them when we slip back into our workaday mental routines. Witnesses to major accidents and violent crimes—events that engender panic and anxiety—tend to forget much of what they saw unless they somehow return to the state of hyperarousal they felt then. Sometimes this happens automatically, when they're in the throes of some unrelated crisis; other times, it's intentionally engineered through coaching or hypnosis. Singers and actors often struggle to recall lines offstage that spring forth automatically when they're performing.

Strictly speaking, state-bound knowledge figures into every aspect of our memory function. Howard Erlichman, a psychologist at the City University of New York, asserts, "The events of the day—a bus splattering mud on you, being yelled at by your boss, or seeing a movie you enjoy—create a cognitive basis that makes some memories more likely to come to mind while others become less probable. Things that make you feel good prime more happy memories, while things that get you down prime sad ones."

In an academic context, state-bound knowledge manifests itself in a host of interesting ways. Consider students who stay awake consuming caffeine or amphetamines so they can cram all night before an exam. The next day, they are likely to forget much of what they studied—not necessarily because they are tired, but because they are not in the same state of mind they were in when they

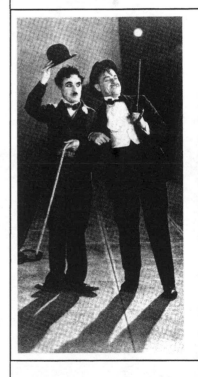

In Chaplin's film *City Lights*, a sober tramp and a drunk millionaire greet a passerby in distinctly different manners. The morning after, the tramp, still sober, recalls the incident; the millionaire, newly sober, does not—until he gets drunk again. This is a perfect example of state-bound knowledge.

studied. One solution, logically, is for students to try as much as possible to coordinate their study time, situation, and state of mind with their anticipated exam time, situation, and state of mind. For example, if the exam is to be given in a classroom during the afternoon, students might try studying for it in a classroom during previous afternoons with the same degree of seriousness as they will most likely have when they actually take it. Consider, also, students who develop the habit of reading certain texts in certain settings: for instance, chemistry books on a commuter train or novels beside a peaceful lake. To recall a text more vividly, these students would do well to invoke the mood or sensations they associate with the corresponding reading environment.

Memory

is fired by association. When we perceive something . . . from that perception we are able to obtain a notion of some other thing like or unlike which is associated with it but has been forgotten.

—Plato

This kind of memory trigger has been invaluable to neuroscientist John Lilly, author of *The Center of the Cyclone* and *The Mind of the Dolphin,* who has made a career out of mapping nonordinary forms of consciousness through isolation-tank and controlled-drug experiments. Continually plagued by the difficulty of recalling what impressed him during an altered state of consciousness after returning to his "normal" state, Lilly devised the following strategy: When something happens during an experiment that he wants to remember, he mentally and/or physically works himself up into a high pitch of excitement to mark the occasion. Depending on the circumstances, he may embroider the event with an elaborate "mind's eye" fantasy or he may scream and dance in celebration. Later, he recalls the excitement, recreates it, and almost always recaptures what it was that so stimulated him.

In our everyday lives, we can take a similar approach. If, for instance, we want to reclaim those grand thoughts we had on vacation, we can try to immerse ourselves in the physical, mental, and/or emotional sensations associated with that vacation. This endeavor may involve eating a special meal, talking with a friend, wearing an outfit, listening to music, looking at photographs, or engaging in a sport that will inspire specific "sense memories" of that vacation. Or it may mean simply sitting back and thinking about the vacation, until our long-lost grand thoughts suddenly and magically return to us.

Why Do We Have Déjà Vu Experiences?

Among the most intriguing phenomena associated with memory is the déjà vu experience (*déjà vu* is French for "already seen"). We encounter a new situation and yet feel we've encountered it before. Frequently the déjà vu experience happens when we're doing something out of the ordinary, like vacationing, house-hunting, or making new acquaintances. But it can also creep up on us when we're engaged in our normal routines. We can walk down a street we've traveled a hundred times before, and, although it's a "new" walk, suddenly it seems as if we've lived through the exact same moment in the forgotten past or in a dream or in another life altogether. We're not terrified, but we're disturbed. Have we simply lost a memory, or have we somehow lost our minds? Are we reconnecting with a past reality, or are we entering the Twilight Zone?

Doctors have discovered that the déjà vu feeling can be artificially triggered by electrical stimulation of the brain's temporal lobe (as can the *jamais vu* or "never seen" feeling, which makes the well-known seem alien to us). This fact has led most experts to believe the déjà vu experience results from an "echo" effect in the brain's processing of information. For some reason, a fresh impression registers in the brain as if it were a recalled memory, with the same general sense of familiarity, completeness, and meaning.

Many cognitive scientists say that when we experience déjà vu, we enter a very mild and short-lived state of mental dissociation. This dissociation could take any one of a number of forms. Maybe we slip into a semi-detached awareness of ourselves being aware of our surroundings, and this double awareness almost instantaneously turns any new sensation into something like a memory. Or perhaps for a few seconds we delay interweaving new information with related material in our memory bank, so that the new information strikes us as mysteriously significant: We understand it, we even feel that in some way we know all about it, but we can't figure out why. This type of "isolated memory consciousness" commonly happens to paranoics or schizophrenics, who can spontaneously read a whole universe of personal meaning into a chance sight, sound, taste, smell, or touch.

A less scientific but equally plausible theory held by many memory experts is that the déjà vu sensation can be aroused whenever a combination of elements in our present experience somehow evokes a specific past experience that our conscious mind cannot identify. Suppose you enter an oak-paneled room for the first time, smell fresh roasted peanuts, and immediately have that tingling, half-trance sensation that you've been there before, that you know all about the place. It's possible that on a similar day in your past (for example, a day when it also rained, a day when you also felt adventurous, a day when you also were sunburned, or a day when you also had breakfast with your sister) you wore similar clothes and for the first time walked into a room that was oak-paneled and suffused with the smell of roasted peanuts.

If the latter explanation is true, our present life may be more pervasively affected by our past memories than we can ever realize or control. The feeling of déjà vu is often linked to the feeling of falling in love. It's quite possible that we get a special sensation around a particular person because that person, or the environment surrounding our meeting of that person, magically evokes haunting sensations of a past, pleasurable event.

One thing is sure about the déjà vu experience—there's nothing we can do about it. It will come when it will come and may or may not influence our subsequent behavior. We can only accept it as a vivid reminder that memory works in mysterious ways. In this respect, we're as helpless as Yogi Berra was at the re-rehiring of Billy Martin to coach the New York Yankees. "Wow," Berra exclaimed, "it's like déjà vu all over again!"

PAST-LIFE RECALL

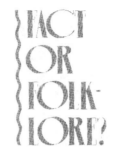

{ FACT OR FOLK- LORE?

According to a 1982 Gallup Poll, 23 percent of Americans believe in reincarnation. Among them are such celebrities as Shirley MacLaine, who recalls a prior existence as a court jester personally beheaded by Louis XV, and Sylvester Stallone, who remembers having been a boxer killed by a knockout in 1935. The majority of Americans, however, remain steadfastly skeptical, as does the Western World in general. Reincarnation flies in the face of scientific logic and Judeo-Christian doctrine. What are respectable Westerners to think about the alleged ability of some apparently sane, intelligent people to recall past lives? What are they to make of the past lives themselves?

From 1946 through 1966, Dr. Ian Stevenson scientifically investigated and documented dozens of episodes of past-life recall. He found that the most rewarding case histories occurred in cultures that support a belief in reincarnation. After all, if a society is not conditioned to acknowledge or respect a particular phenomenon, it is not likely to provide fruitful evidence relating to that phenomenon. He also developed a preference for interviewing children, since their memories of past lives proved to be fresher, less prejudiced, and easier to evaluate.

One of the most provocative stories in Stevenson's 1966 study, *Twenty Cases Suggestive of Reincarnation,* involves Shanti Devi, born in Delhi, India, in 1926. At the age of seven, Shanti announced to her parents that she had lived previously in the distant town of Muttra as a woman named Ludgi and had died ten years ago giving birth to her third child. Shanti's relatives and neighbors kept track of the many details she recounted but made no attempt to verify them. Several years later, a man came to her house for the first time on business, and she welcomed him as her "former" husband's cousin. The flabbergasted visitor revealed that he was from Muttra and did have a cousin who had lost a wife named Ludgi in childbirth during the year in question. Later, he arranged for his cousin to cross

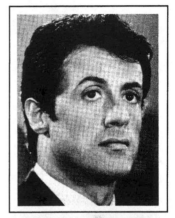

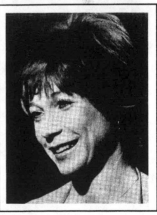

Perhaps playing many roles in their present lifetimes has helped actors Sylvester Stallone and Shirley MacLaine to recall previous roles in previous lifetimes.

Shanti's path as if by chance, and she immediately greeted him as her past husband. Her parents then took her to Muttra, where witnesses confirm that she correctly pointed out directions and buildings (often while being led blindfolded through the streets), identified Ludgi's first two children (but, understandably, not the third), and actually spoke to Ludgi's relatives in the local dialect, to which she had never been exposed in her present lifetime!

Stevenson declines to speculate on the meaning of Shanti's story or of past-life histories in general. By contrast, modern-day Western practitioners of past-life therapy, be they accredited psychiatrists or entrepreneurial laypeople, claim that knowledge of one's past lives can have enormous practical value in terms of resolving one's present-life problems. Typically, past-life regression is facilitated by simple hypnotic suggestion (see "Fact or Folklore?: Hypnotic Trance," page 54). Some therapists also advise their clients to perform daily meditation exercises designed to transport the mind back through time and to sharpen recall of "value-laden" images. Once a client has established the nature of a given past life, then he or she can begin tracing ways in which that past life may be influencing his or her present life. If you have a fear of flying, for example, it may be due to a bad flying or falling experience you had in a previous life. Are you irrationally and perpetually angry at your mother? Maybe it's because of abuse you suffered at a "former" mother's hands.

For believers in reincarnation, past-life therapy seems to work amazingly well. Nonbelievers explain this as a placebo effect: If you think something is going to work, then it has a better chance of working; and having any systematic explanation for the cause of a malady helps one to work on overcoming the malady. But how are nonbelievers to account for the past-life memories themselves? Assuming fraud isn't a factor, where do they come from? Some authorities insist that the past-life recaller is merely confusing a strikingly vivid hallucination (possibly suggested by a book or a movie) with a past-life memory. Others propose that a form of ESP is at work, that the subject is telepathically or clairvoyantly picking up information from another source. Still others suggest the subject may be plumbing a "genetic" memory system made up of inherited images associated either with his or her direct ancestors or with the human race as a whole.

Often the subject of purported past-life recall has been shown to be a victim of cryptomnesia. A cryptomnesiac accesses previously absorbed information that has been forgotten and, mistakenly but genuinely, feels this information is part of his or her personal experience. In the 1960s, Dr. Reina Kaupman, a Finnish psychiatrist, assisted a student, through hypnosis, to uncover a past life as a thirteenth-century English girl named Dorothy. The student even sang a folk song in Middle English, a language she'd never studied. In a later hypnotic session, Kaupman regressed the student to the age of thirteen in her present life. Among her memories of that year was a time when she picked up a book in a library and idly flipped through the pages for a minute or two. She remembered (literally, she saw) that the authors were Benjamin Britten and Imogen Holst. With considerable effort, Kaupman found the book, and there was the folk song— with Middle English lyrics.

We may not be able to prove that reincarnation exists, but we also can't prove that it doesn't exist. Dr. Shelby Carver of the University of Chicago comments, "How *would* you go about constructing a reliable proof for reincarnation? Given the mysteries of life and the human mind, past lives are certainly within the realm of possibility." If past-life recall is possible, then why not future-life recall? As the White Queen says to Alice in Lewis Carroll's *Through the Looking-Glass,* "It's a poor sort of memory that works only backwards."

Will My Memory Powers Decline As I Get Older?

Grandpa sits on the porch swing, reliving the morning when he and 300 other GIs liberated Naples. He can still see the flowers that pretty Italian girl gave him and hear the spirited march played by the Army band. Suddenly an infant cries, and his thoughts snap forward to the present. There in the playpen before him, struggling to stand, is his one-year-old grandson. Just now, Grandpa can't recall his name. Meanwhile, his grandson is absorbing every detail of Grandpa's puzzled face, the swing, and the quality of light and air on the porch. Ten years from now, however, he'll be lucky to remember any image from his life before the age of three.

Our state of memory definitely changes depending on our stage of life, but it can't be said that any new state is significantly better or worse than another. Older people *appear* to forget things more easily, but—assuming they are mentally healthy (which is a safe assumption 80 percent of the time)—this is largely because older people have more to remember. As we age, the amount of information in our memory banks increases, but the percentage we can recall easily stays the same. Short-term memory operations do slow down a bit, but they are no less accurate or complete; and the tradeoff is deeper and richer long-term memories.

Grandpa remembers liberating Naples more clearly than he does his new grandson's name because the Naples memory has had more time to "consolidate," or weave webs of associative connections with other memory data. It's more likely that his memory will lead him to this major turning point in his life than to the newly established name of his grandson. This doesn't mean his grandson isn't important to him as a person. He just doesn't have a sufficient motive to remember the name. After all, his grandson can't even recognize it yet!

> *The memory*
> *strengthens as you lay burdens upon it, and becomes*
> *trustworthy as you trust it.*
> —Thomas De Quincey

Dr. Cameron Camp, a psychologist at the University of New Orleans, believes that many of the memory "defects" older people exhibit are the result of practical decisions—conscious or not—about what can afford to be forgotten (at least temporarily) and what can't. "Older adults may generate more 'forget' cues," he speculates, noting that older people are less apt to encounter truly "new"—that is, "memorable"—information and are more willing to forego keeping track of "nonmemorable" details. "The ability to forget some previously learned information may allow older adults to focus on underlying principles," Camp says.

Names, like phone numbers, dates, and other "tag-pieces" of information, are prime targets for acquired for-getfulness. We may do better at remembering names when we're twenty-five than we did when we were fif-teen, thanks to greater social and professional demands, but typically we do worse at thirty-five than we did at twenty-five, worse at forty-five than we did at thirty-five, and so on.

As for the opposite end of the age spectrum, theories abound to explain why we remember so little, if anything, about the obviously novel and impressive years between birth and age three. Freud posited that a young child's thoughts are so incestuous and violent that he or she later suppresses them. Since Freud, psychologists are more in-clined to attribute "infantile amnesia" to the huge discrep-ancy between our world view from birth to three—when we lack physical authority, verbal skill, and discriminating judgment—and our world view thereafter (see "Words for the Wise: State-Bound Knowledge," page 84). Preceding all these theories is the fact that the hippocampus, the brain structure necessary for conscious memory, is not fully developed until age one and a half or two.

At each stage along the age spectrum after childhood, we remember certain parts of our lives far more easily than oth-ers, depending on the image we have of ourselves or our personal needs at that stage. For example, most people around age fifty recall their early twenties in more detail than they recall their thirties and early forties. Facing the onset of "old age," they spend more time reviving memories of the years when they first began defining themselves as

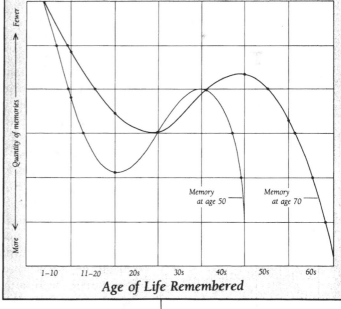

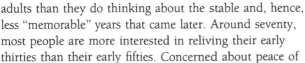

Age of Life Remembered

adults than they do thinking about the stable and, hence, less "memorable" years that came later. Around seventy, most people are more interested in reliving their early thirties than their early fifties. Concerned about peace of mind, they work on remembering the era when they first sensed they were in their "stable" prime.

Autobiographical memories, of course, are highly subject to screening. We can easily forget those parts of our lives that we don't want to remember and highlight those parts that we do. We can also warp certain memories to suit later purposes, and conveniently forget that we've done so. In a recent follow-up study of 310 middle-aged men and women who had been treated as children in the same guidance clinic, researchers established that those who were well-adjusted in their present life had fewer memories of the painful events in their childhood than did those who were currently suffering from emotional problems. In another study, mothers were asked to recall when their children had reached important developmental milestones. Their answers proved to be earlier or later than the actual dates, corresponding to what they had come to believe was preferable from child-rearing authorities.

To maintain a "true" and productive memory of each of life's stages, the following activities are recommended.

• Keep a daily or weekly journal. Record not only details of what happens—names, places, and events—but also general impressions regarding your thoughts and feelings. It will not only refresh your memory of the past as you grow older, but also get you into the habit of observing your present more intently and constructively.
• Every now and then, put yourself in the shoes of a younger or older person. You can imagine you are yourself at another age, someone you know who is older or younger, or simply "Person X" who is older or younger. Then act your imaginary age. If you want to recapture what it feels like—and felt like—to be a child, for example, try crawling around the floor and seeing things from a child's height. If you want to anticipate what might interest you about your present life when you're older, pretend you're at the close of your life dictating your memoirs to a secretary.
• Regularly question your past and your future. Compare your personal memories of your childhood with those of other family members or with those of people who lived in your neighborhood while you were growing up.

When confronted with a present challenge, think about how you would have handled it—for good or for ill—five years ago. When contemplating the future, ask yourself, "What do I want my life to be like five years from now?" and be as specific in your response as you can

❖❖❖❖❖❖❖❖❖❖

Everyone
complains of his memory, but no one complains of his judgment.
—Duc François de La Rochefoucauld

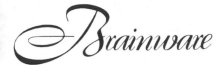

Psion Organizer II

Undeniably the most useful external memory aid is one that can accompany you wherever you go throughout the day. After all, a brainstorm, an interesting bit of knowledge, a propitious worktime, or a need-to-know situation can pop up at any moment. When that moment strikes, don't rely on a three-by-five notepad or a mini-tape-recorder tucked into your pocket. Instead, reach for the Psion Organizer II: an 8.8-ounce, handheld device that functions as a combination computer, calculator, writing desk, and filing system. Especially convenient for the traveler, it can unobtrusively access information, record important data, check your schedule, and perform computations while you're standing in line for a plane, or talking on the phone, or sitting in a meeting, or downing a beer at a crowded bar. Attach a special linkup, and you can also transfer what your Psion Organizer II remembers directly to another computer back home or at the office.

```
┌──────────────────────Daily Calendar──────────────────────┐
│ EVIN    Evin Ollinger              Wednesday  6/01/88  8:00 am │
├───────────────────────────────────────────────────────────┤
│ 8am.  9  .  10 .  11  .  Noon  1pm.  2  .  3  .  4  .  5  .  6  .  7  .  8pm │
├──────────────────────────────────────────────────────────┤
 WHEN──────WHO──────WHAT──────DESCRIPTION──────
  8:00a   Others-?  R&D:       Meeting to discuss new products:
 10:00a   Me/us?    R&D        Who/What/When Office (LAN), OS/2
 10:30a ! CINDY     PRINTJOB:  Call to discuss advertising schedule
 11:00a   Others    BROCHURE:  Meeting to discuss new brochure
 12:00a
 12:30p   Others    R&D:       Lunch:  Continue discussion of Who/What/When
  2:00p                        Office (LAN) and OS/2
  3:00p   MARY T    FLYER:     Assign layout for flyer/discuss deadlines
  4:00p
 TO:DO  A GREG      R&D:       Call to discuss connectivity
 TO:DO  B                      Review sales strategy goals
 TO:DO  C           BUDGET:    MILESTONE: Development budget
                               Review development budget
 TO:DO  D BOB C     SALES:     Receive and review quarterly Sales Report
                               (Follow Up)
```

Use the arrow keys to select tasks for editing. Press "Ins" to add new tasks.
F1=Help F2=Calendar F3=Dial F4=Memo F6=Top F7=Prev F8=Next F10=Save ESC=Quit

Hypertext Programs

The sharply defined, single-access way in which the computer stores data in its memory differs radically from the associative, multi-access way in which the brain stores data in its memory. Now there's a whole new category of software known as hypertext programs that makes it easier for the brain's memory to work with the computer's memory. Operating a hypertext program, for example, you only have to press a key to connect individual calendar entries to all the relevant information in your computer files. If you need to write a certain business report or meet with a specific client, you can quickly call up a list of pertinent files and even use significant words and phrases to locate smaller units of material scattered throughout your data base. Enormous times-savers, these programs also prevent you from inadvertently consigning valuable facts and figures to oblivion simply because you've forgotten the proper file title and/or the detailed contents of individual files.

Shoebox I Plus

The computer revolution has worked small miracles in assisting people to jog their memories—especially when it comes to keeping track of daily tasks, needs, and obligations. Among the most recent and impressive software programs designed to put your brain on top of your schedule is Shoebox I Plus, a product of R & R Associates Inc. Its primary component is a calendar that expands and contracts to fit the volume of data it contains. The program also offers "reminder flags" that can be automatically situated at regular intervals up to three months in the future, saving you the trouble of making separate, repetitive entries. Other features include a search option that tells you immediately what time blocks remain open in a given week, month, or quarter-year and an expense-tracking function that delivers a day-by-day budget status. With a hard disk, you can call the Shoebox I Plus program on-screen for quick reference or updating even while you're in the midst of another program.

```
┌────────────────────────────────────────────────────────────┐
│ SHOEBOX          Appointments for George Arno    Tuesday 08/08/89 │
│═════════════════════════════════════════════════════════════│
│  Time/Date   Description                              9:18a  │
│═════════════════════════════════════════════════════════════│
│   8:00a      _____                                     │
│   9:00a      _____                                     │
│  10:00a      _____                                     │
│  11:00a      _____                                     │
│  12:00n- 2:00p Kiwanis Luncheon at Hotel Intown              │
│   2:00p      _____                                     │
│   3:00p      _____         ═══════════════════════     │
│   4:00p      _____              August 1989            │
│                                  ═══════════════════════     │
│                                   S  M  T  W  T  F  S        │
│                                  ═══════════════════════     │
│                                  30 31  1  2  3  4  5        │
│                                   6  7  8  9 10 11 12        │
│                                  13 14 15 16 17 18 19        │
│                                  20 21 22 23 24 25 26        │
│                                  27 28 29 30 31  1  2        │
│                                   3  4  5  6  7  8  9        │
│═════════════════════════════════════════════════════════════│
│  *** To begin enter command code from below or press ? for explanations *** │
│  ? Help!  B Brief   C Change   D Another Day  E Expenses  F Find  H History │
│  N New appointment  O Other    P Print    Q Quit    R Reminders │
└────────────────────────────────────────────────────────────┘
```

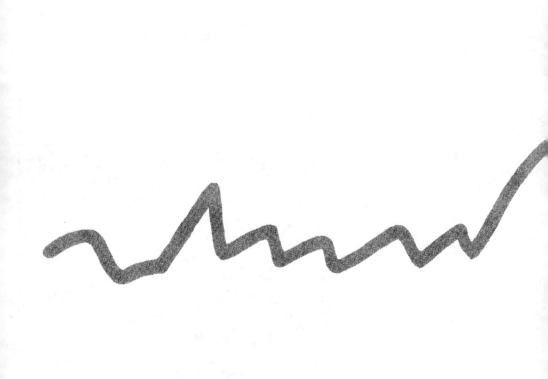

4
INTELLIGENCE

Rumor has it that we use only 10 percent of our brain's intellectual capacity. In reality, this statistic is meaningless—except as an indicator of the fact that we are far from knowing the limits of the mind's capabilities.

The brain's intellectual activity is not a percentage game. Huge sections of the brain can suffer damage without any apparent long-term effects on the victim's intelligence or behavior. Damage to certain tiny areas, however, can be disastrous on both scores. Electrical stimulation of a single neuron activates hundreds of "information bits," but even the simplest thought requires unknown millions of neurons to process. For all we know, there isn't a single part of our brain that doesn't get used sometime, somehow; yet this doesn't

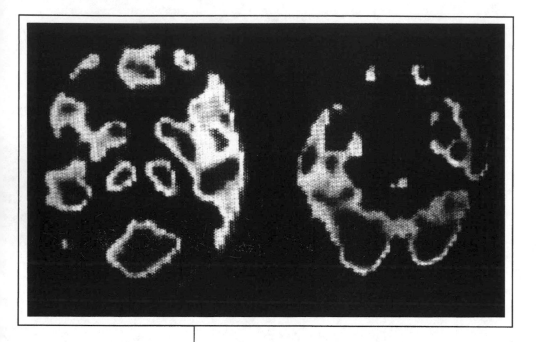

Here we have two different PET scans of a thinking brain—specifically, the brain of a man listening to a Sherlock Holmes mystery and trying to solve it. Both images represent neurochemical activity at the same moment in time. The image on the left was made at a higher level of the brain's cerebrum than the image on the right. (For more information on PET scanners, see page 30.)

mean that any one of these parts is necessarily indispensable, permanent, or functioning to its full potential.

One article of popular wisdom about the brain's intelligence is unarguably true: Use it or lose it. The renowned neurologist Dr. Gardner Murphy states this principle more scientifically: "Uncultivated cortical functions diminish in strength when they are not used, much as muscles weaken when they are not exercised." Given regular workouts, our intelligence grows ever more powerful, more flexible, and more agile. Without such challenges, our intelligence rapidly weakens.

Experiments conducted with animals over the past twenty years suggest that the structure of cells in the brain's cortex physically changes as a result of sustained intellectual exercise, with individual neurons developing more connective links (dendritic branches) to other neurons, and gray matter as a whole becoming thicker and denser. Assuming what's true of rat brains is also true of human brains, each person plays a significant role in the literal creation of his or her brain stuff.

How, then do we go about the business of exercising our intelligence? The first and most important step is to appreciate that intelligence takes many forms and, therefore, that keeping our intelligence in shape calls for many different types of exercise. Dr. Howard Gardner, a Harvard psychologist, divides intelligence into seven different categories.

1. *Linguistic skills*
   - facility in writing and reading, speaking and listening to speech
   - involves understanding verbal tones and shadings as well as the definitions and connotations of individual words
   - especially important to authors, philosophers, and journalists
2. *Logical–mathematical skills*
   - facility in analysis and calculation, problem-solving, and decision-making
   - the skill area most emphasized in formal education and testing
   - especially important to scientists and business people
3. *Musical skills*
   - facility in melodic and harmonic expression
   - primarily involves producing music, but also involves listening to music and reading music
   - especially important to singers and instrumentalists
4. *Spatial skills*
   - facility in working with forms, shapes, and perspectives
   - involves imagining spatial possibilities as well as physically designing spaces

On the left is a neuron with relatively few dendritic branches. On the right is a neuron with an abundance of dendritic branches, which can result from long-term exposure to intellectual challenges.

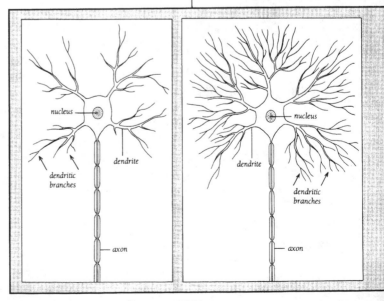

- especially important to painters, architects, and urban planners
5. *Bodily and kinesthetic skills*
   - facility in movement and handling objects
   - involves coordinated physical and mental control
   - especially important to dancers, athletes, and surgeons
6. *Interpersonal skills*
   - facility in interpreting, affecting, and managing the behavior of others
   - a highly comprehensive skill area, closely linked to many of the other six forms of intelligence
   - especially important to salespeople and politicians
7. *Intrapersonal skills*
   - facility in understanding one's own inner nature and the inner nature of others
   - involves developing self-awareness, intuition, and empathy
   - especially important to psychologists and spiritual leaders

Most of us utilize all of these intellectual skills in the course of our lives, but very few of us draw on each of these skills to the same extent. We specialize, and this, too, influences the way our physical brain takes shape. With the aid of fine-focus optical devices, Dr. Arnold Scheibel, director of UCLA's Brain Research Institute, peers into the brains of people having different professions, and what he has seen is, in a word, mind-blowing. The cortex of a typist's brain, for example, had longer and more complex neurons than average in the region governing finger movement. In the case of a musician, the cortex was more developed around the area responsible for sound-processing.

We can't expect ourselves to give equal attention to every one of the seven intellectual skills mentioned above, so that our brain is, in an almost literal sense, "well-rounded." But we can take it upon ourselves to make sure no one skill gets completely ignored. When this happens, a whole dimension of our intelligence languishes and, in time, withers away.

Our day-to-day life inevitably offers a fair amount of intellectual exercise, but with very little effort we can give our brain a much richer intellectual environment. It's

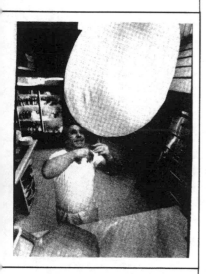

"Intelligence" is often confused with "book smarts." While linguistic skills and logical–mathematical skills are definitely forms of intelligence, so are other skills, such as the ability to perform feats of physical coordination.

partly a matter of attitude: for instance, being a more alert observer of the world around us, taking our ambitions more seriously, and looking for lessons in our daily experience. It's also partly a matter of enterprise, which means taking the time and expending the energy to do things that will help boost our intelligence.

The articles in this chapter will help you design and set up your own customized mental exercise program, so that you can make the most effective and creative use of your intelligence. You'll also learn more about the wide variety of possible intellectual capacities: from youth through old age, from so-called "idiot" savants to geniuses. And you'll discover what kinds of tests work—or don't work—to measure your basic intelligence quotient; what kinds of meals do—or don't—provide food for thought; and what kinds of brain machines may—or may not—be smart buys.

What Are the Best Ways to Increase My Intelligence?

Common sense tells us that the primary resource for intelligence on intelligence is the education field. It so happens that the last few years have been revolutionary ones in the classroom. Faced with a rapidly escalating increase in the diversity of students, the complexity of subject matter, and the competitiveness of the job market that awaits its graduates, the American school system has been forced to rethink its strategy. What it has taught itself is worth teaching ourselves. Here, in the educational field's own jargon, are suggestions for making the brain brighter.

Practice Critical Reasoning. Concerned about turning out students that are truly intelligent rather than simply knowledgeable, educators are restructuring the way they approach subject matter in the classroom. Instead of getting their students to memorize facts and deliver "right" answers, they're providing their students with "problem-rich" situations and then turning them loose to explore these situations with their own critical reasoning.

In a math class, for example, the critical reasoning project may be a school census. Involved in planning that census would be all sorts of brain-building challenges: What possible things could the census reveal? How could it be designed so it would yield that information? What are various possible sampling, distribution, and calculation procedures? What are the time and resource logistics for each procedure? As they work out the census, the math students pick up the basic math skills they need. Thus, the skills become means to an end, which makes them far easier and more interesting to learn than if they were an end in themselves.

You can practice critical reasoning in your own life by setting an ambitious goal for yourself and then figuring out all the steps you might take, and the time and resources you might need, to fulfill that goal. Whether it's mastering a foreign language so you can travel with more pleasure, remodeling your basement so you have more room to entertain, or assembling a family history for your children so they can pass it along to their children, the project should ideally be something that intrigues you, that is full of practical possibilities, and that ties in with many different facets of your life. You might even try helping kids with their homework and school projects: It's an excellent way to combine learning with togetherness.

Write Across the Curricula. Why were we compelled by our English teachers to write so many essays? With extremely rare exceptions, it was not so that the world might benefit from our impressions of *The Scarlet Letter* or from a frank exposé of our summer vacation. Essays were required because the essay-writing activity itself gives the writer practice in applying clarity, logic, organization, and development to his or her thoughts, and, best of all, it reveals *how* (as well as *what*) the writer thinks.

Today, essays in school are no longer confined to English class. Recognizing that essay-writing functions as an excellent means of learning how to think better, teachers are working it into every subject area (hence the phrase "writing across the curricula").

You can do the same thing for the same purpose in

your present, nonacademic life. Record daily discoveries in a journal. Write your way through a difficult decision-making process. Beef up your correspondence. Invent tales for your children. And just for the health of it, assign yourself topics of interest to discuss in writing.

Broaden the Dialogue. In the classroom, "broadening the dialogue" refers to creating more—and different—interpersonal teaching and learning relationships. Students may be called upon to instruct the teacher about something he or she might not know. Rotating shifts of students may work together on different projects. Outside experts may be brought into the classroom to speak, or students may go outside the classroom to interview experts. The idea is that the more various the minds with which a student comes into contact, the more enlightened the student's own mind will be.

Try "broadening the dialogue" among your own circle of friends, relatives, and acquaintances. Seek as many different opinions on a specific matter as you can get. Form "buddy" relationships for certain types of multifaceted, intellectually demanding situations (like writing business reports, or learning a new sport, or repairing your car). Always be on the lookout for situations or events that will expand your number of contacts.

Cultivate Mentally Enriching Extracurricular Activities. An extracurricular activity, inside or outside the classroom, is something that you do strictly for entertainment; but if it can be educational as well, so much the better. Reading ranks high on any list of intellectually stimulating leisure-time activities, especially if it involves "cross-discipline" reading: not exclusively fiction or nonfiction, science or art, popular works or scholarly works, but a mixture of all of these.

Other recurring items on such lists include: sketching; painting; photography; visiting museums; completing crossword puzzles; playing board games that require word-building, drawing, or planning skills; maintaining a collection; bird- or animal-watching. Again, involving mates, kids, or friends in your brain-building endeavors doubles the learning and the fun.

From Bonehead to Conehead

During the Middle Ages, the conical cap was the brain machine of choice. Invented by the philosopher Duns Scotus, it supposedly contained and intensified the brain's energy—a sort of "pyramid-power" in reverse. Quickly associated with witches, wizards, and professional sages, it was also fashionably adapted by ladies at court, who hoped it might help them make up for their alleged intellectual inferiority to men. The Duns cap survived into the twentieth century as the dunce cap. No longer seriously considered a means of making people smarter or more attractive, it was used to identify and embarrass poor students, so that they would strive to avoid ever having to wear it again.

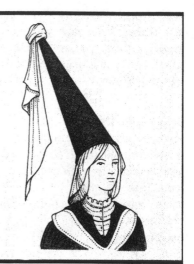

GENIUS

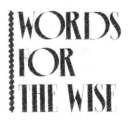

Few terms are more loosely applied than "genius." Scientists define a genius as a person having an IQ above 140 (less than one percent of the population). But to the world at large, a genius is as a genius does. Assuming you display exceptional "braininess" on a fairly consistent basis, you can be a genius in the laboratory, in the boardroom, in the kitchen, on the basketball court, wherever, even though your IQ is an average 100. By the same token, you can have an IQ of 180 and schlump through life with nary a clever thought or deed.

If it isn't one's IQ that makes one a genius, what does? To date, the search for a physical cause of genius has proved fruitless. Certainly the size of the brain has nothing to do with it. The average brain weighs between forty-four and forty-nine ounces; the brains of widely acclaimed geniuses have in some cases weighed more (like the English poet Lord Byron's brain at 82.25 ounces); in some cases, less (like the French writer Anatole France's brain at 35 ounces); but in most cases, the same.

Studies of cortical formations (the ridge-and-groove pattern on the brain's surface) have also failed miserably. In 1925, the Soviet Union entrusted Lenin's brain to the German neurologist Oskar Vogt with the goal, according to Vogt's psychiatric colleague Walter Reich, of establishing "an institute in Moscow entirely devoted to the purpose of discovering the 'materialist' (that is, 'physical') basis for Lenin's political and philosophical genius." The institute itself never materialized. In California, neuroscientists are still studying slices of Einstein's brain in the hope of finding a physical explanation for genius, but they've had no more luck than their Leninist counterparts.

Others seek the origins of genius in heredity. Perhaps, they theorize, certain combinations of genetic traits—whether they be related directly to intelligence or not—produce the necessary "smarts" for genius. There's no progress to report on this front, either, but that hasn't

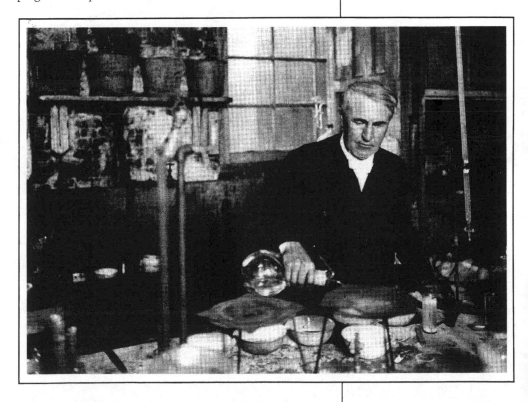

In a 1988 poll of college students, Thomas Edison was most often identified as "the leading genius in American history."

discouraged Robert Graham, an American multimillionaire and philanthropist. Firmly convinced that the secret behind genius does involve a high IQ, Frank has established a "genius sperm bank," officially called Repository for Germinal Choice, in Escondido, California. Inside its offices, women desirous of bearing genius offspring can peruse the histories of hundreds of volunteer sperm donors, all of whom had to have an IQ score over 140 to donate. There are no guarantees, of course. There are also no IQ qualifications for sperm recipients.

Yet another die-hard speculation is that genius issues from madness, neurosis, or disability (real or perceived). In this respect, great achievements are deemed compensatory acts. Vincent Van Gogh's idiosyncratic painting style is viewed as a direct expression of the mental turmoil that ultimately drove him insane. Winston Churchill's need to focus his pathological hostility on an outside enemy is credited for his outstanding moral leadership in the struggle against Hitler's Germany. Sylvia Plath's manic-depressive personality is held equally responsible for her emotionally charged poetry and for her death by suicide. Napoleon Bonaparte is said to have sought stature as a military hero because he lacked stature as a physical being. Intriguing as such connections may be, they can't be proven, nor can significant patterns of madness, neurosis, or disability be drawn among large groups of geniuses as opposed to large groups of non-geniuses.

The most convincing theories about what causes genius come from the gifted horses' mouths. Whether exceptional athletes, extraordinary musicians, or inspired scientists, publicly accredited geniuses cite the same determining factors.

Early Encouragement. If the strong intellectual drive associated with childhood can be nurtured so that it stays with the individual child as he or she matures, the chances are much greater that the ensuing adult will perform feats of genius. Particularly valuable are youthful "apprenticeship" relationships. An older mentor introduced Swedish film director Ingmar Bergman to the intricacies of the magic lantern when Bergman was still a child; Margaret Drabble, the English novelist, grew up in a family that read together; James Baldwin, the American writer, traced his success to the extracurricular coaching of a favorite elementary school teacher.

Hard Work. Geniuses tend to be almost hyperactive in comparison to the general population. They derive primary satisfaction in life from their personal productivity. Therefore, it is not surprising that they're inclined to invent a major portion of their job, whether they work alone or in a large organization offering clearly defined job descriptions. With such a big stake in doing well, they are unusually committed and diligent. Hence we have the expression commonly attributed to American inventor Thomas Edison: "Genius is 10 percent inspiration, 90 percent perspiration."

Rudyard Kipling, the English poet, short-story writer, and novelist, frequently lectured on the positive contributions of good diet, daily exercise, and travel to the development of "a genius mentality."

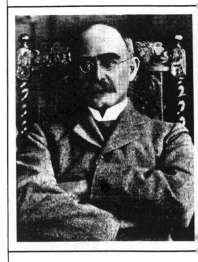

Faith. Contrary to many people's image of the genius as a tormented pessimist, most geniuses harbor positive attitudes toward their work and their chances of success. Typically, they invest a great deal of faith in a higher force. Giacomo Puccini, the Italian composer, called this force Omnipotence and God: "The secret of all creative geniuses is that they possess the power to appropriate the beauty, the wealth, the grandeur, and the sublimity within their own souls, which are a part of Omnipotence, and to communicate those riches to others. . . . The music [of *Madame Butterfly*] was dictated to me by God; I was merely instrumental in putting it on paper and communicating it to the public." The English writer Rudyard Kipling called this higher force his Personal Daemon: "Let us now consider the Personal Daemon. . . . Most men, and some most unlikely, keep him under an alias which varies with their literary or scientific attainments. Mine came to me early when I sat bewildered among other notions, and said, 'Take this and no other.' I obeyed, and was rewarded. . . . When your Daemon is in charge, do not try to think consciously. Drift, wait, and obey. . . ."

How Well Do Standardized Tests Measure the Brain's Intelligence?

Shortly after World War I, the French Minister of Public Education hired Dr. Alfred Binet, a renowned psychologist, to develop a means of identifying children with special learning needs. The result was, in English terms, the first intelligence quotient or IQ test. Quickly it evolved into the primary instrument used in schools and businesses throughout the world to rate the taker's basic, "fixed" intellectual powers: a score between 85 and 115 denoting average intelligence; above 115, high intelligence; and below 85, low intelligence. Now over 200 varieties of IQ tests exist, each using the same scale. The most familiar models in the United States are the Stanford-Binet Intelligence Quotient Test (for children under twelve) and the Wechsler Adult Intelligence Scale (for adolescents and adults).

Strangely enough, widespread official acceptance of the IQ test has never stopped it from being highly controversial. Debate among scientific and educational experts has continued to swirl around two principal questions: (1) In what sense is a person's basic intelligence a "fixed" entity—one that remains stable from childhood onward? (2) Does the IQ test itself accurately reflect a taker's basic intelligence?

At least by the age of five or six, when we begin our formal schooling and are most likely to take our first (and, often, only) IQ test, it does appear that we possess a "basic" intellectual facility that is as permanent a part of who we are as our "basic" personality. While we can possibly score higher or lower on subsequent IQ tests, the typical experience in such cases suggest that our score won't change much. We can increase our knowledge, sharpen our problem-solving skills, and learn to express ourselves more creatively at each different stage in our life, but our intellectual "equipment," as it were, remains the same.

What, then, is responsible for this equipment? Do we inherit it from our forebears? Do we build it from our surroundings during those first critical years of brain/mind development? Or does it come to us as a freak of fate? Since no one knows, we can only assume that any, all, or none of the above possibilities may be responsible. A series of studies made during the 1980s, however, supports the notion that an individual brain's innate processing capability determines its owner's basic intelligence level. By comparing subjects' IQ scores to the results of laboratory tests in which they were asked to signal their first awareness of various tones and lights, researchers have repeatedly demonstrated that the greater the IQ, the less time it takes to process stimuli. The natural conclusion, they argue, is that people with higher intelligence are blessed from birth with more swiftly and smoothly working electrochemical connections between brain cells.

A more serious issue to educators is whether IQ tests are an accurate measure of the taker's basic intelligence. Few critics can justifiably complain that IQ tests lack practical value in fulfilling their orginally intended purpose. The tests do not seem capable of targeting children who require special education, based on achieving scores significantly higher or lower than the norm. On the other hand, few advocates of IQ tests can justifiably claim that the tests are reliable indicators of who's smarter than who within a twenty-point range. The most hotly debated argument concerns whether the tests are comprehensive enough: Do they cover a sufficiently wide range of intellectual skills to be considered arbiters of one's "intelligence quotient"?

Advocates of IQ tests admit that the emphasis in current tests is almost solely on computation and logic, but they insist that these core areas are the most critical in academic and professional performance. Critics disagree, saying that *divergent* intelligence (the ability to speculate and create) is just as important, if not more important, than *convergent* intelligence (the ability to calculate and deduce); therefore, they maintain, IQ tests should measure both forms of intelligence instead of solely the latter.

Another bone of contention is how unfairly IQ tests are biased in favor of the domant cultural group—which, in the United States, means white males from the middle and upper economic classes. Everyone agrees that *some* degree of bias has been inadvertently built into the American tests. When faced with the analogy puzzle "plate is to placemat as cup is to [fill in the blank]," ghetto-dwelling blacks are bound to have more trouble answering "saucer" than suburban-dwelling whites; and it isn't because blacks or lower-class individuals have less basic intelligence. Females in general tend to be penalized by the large percentage of questions dealing with images or facts related to the worlds of sports, mathematics, and science, worlds that the American culture passively—though sometimes actively—discourages females from entering.

The same problems that bedevil IQ tests also plague other standardized intelligence tests, such as the Scholastic Aptitude Test (SAT) and American College Test (ACT). Separately or in combination, the SAT and ACT are taken by over 3 million college applicants each year, and the resulting scores are used as a critical basis for determining who gets admitted to schools and who doesn't. Instead of measuring basic intelligence, they measure acquired knowledge (which means you can prime your score by studying), but, like the IQ test, they focus almost exclusively on convergent, logical thinking at the expense of divergent, creative thinking, and they are inevitably somewhat biased in favor of white males with a middle- or upper-class background.

The solution, at once logical and creative, is to rework all these tests so that they are more comprehensive and less biased. IQ tests designers have been churning out new, improved models for the past fifteen years. In 1989, the ACT completed its first major overhaul since 1959 and unveiled a prototype test that puts more emphasis on essay-style questions (whose answers can be judged for their ingenuity, organization, and style as well as for their "rightness") and more prose passages and charts that require interpretation rather than "solution." Also in 1989, the SAT began a three-year study to improve its content and format. Both the ACT and the SAT development teams have set up ongoing expert panels to weed out any discernible racist, sexist, or elitist biases.

No matter how they're upgraded, IQ tests and other standardized intelligence tests will always be crude instruments for measuring an individual's "basic intelligence." At best, we can only make sure that they're not rude instruments as well. Their limitations should always be recognized, and they should never be used as the only criteria for determining one's capacity to handle a class, a job, or a tough situation.

NO FOOL LIKE AN OLD FOOL

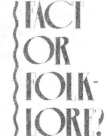

The wise sage or the doddering geezer: which of these two images more accurately reflects what we can expect in old age? Until recently, authorities told us that the brain's intellectual capabilities began deteriorating around age sixty. Now studies are telling the authorities that this isn't true. Tests have shown the brain to be capable of intellectual growth throughout its lifetime. Whether or not our personal brain experiences that growth depends on our individual style of living.

Scientists used to think brain cells went through a great dying-off process in late adulthood, rather like the sloughing of hair follicles. It is a conveniently cautionary myth—just like the myth that alcohol kills brain cells— but the fact is that the only time in the brain's normal life history that it undergoes massive cell loss is early in childhood, after it has succeeded in developing all of its basic physical structures. From that stage onward until late in the eighties (barring illness, accident, or extreme abuse), the brain experiences the same level of metabolic activity and suffers no impairing loss of intelligence.

Some minor aspects of intellectual functioning do seem to diminish around age sixty. Occasionally, mental processing in older people's brains may be fractionally slower than it normally is, and declining vision or hearing may mechanically impede their comprehension or responsiveness. Even if their brains are not experiencing any physical problems, lack of a proper incentive may prevent them from exhibiting how smart they are. These setbacks, however, are frequently accompanied by gains. According to psychologist Jan Sinnott, there are many ways in which an older brain is noticeably superior to a younger one. Sinnott cites the example of an older typist who becomes so experienced at reading ahead in the text that it more than compensates for a decline in typing proficiency. In addition to such clever compensating activities, older people tend to be better than younger people at determining

Prime Time

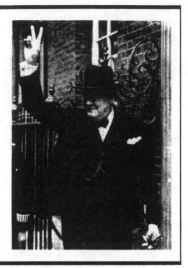

Among countless individuals who have achieved their greatest intellectual triumphs late in life is the British statesman and author Sir Winston Churchill. In 1940, at the age of sixty-four, he became Prime Minister and performed outstanding service to his country and the Allied powers throughout World War II. In 1951, at the age of seventy-five, he was once again chosen to be Prime Minister and fulfilled his duties with admirable skill until his retirement in 1955.

future needs, planning to meet deadlines, and solving problems that rely more on judgment than logic. In short, older brains do test out as wiser brains.

Many gerontologists draw a distinction between "fluid intelligence" and "crystallized intelligence" when they talk about the intellectual capacities of younger people versus older people. Fluid intelligence, at which people from ages fifteen to forty excel, refers to seeing and using abstract relationships and patterns. It comes in handy for calculating, engineering, or playing chess and characteristically wanes in importance for the individual over sixty. Crystallized intelligence, by contrast, involves drawing on an accumulated body of knowledge to make decisions and form opinions. It continues to be prized and nurtured—and, therefore, keeps on improving—throughout old age.

On conventional intelligence tests, older people usually fare slightly worse than younger people, but this is generally due to the nature of the tests themselves. "Many tests that are used to assess the cognitive abilities of the elderly are biased in favor of younger people with whom they are compared," notes Leonard Poon, a psychologist at Harvard University. "One test involved remembering pairs of nonsense words. College students are motivated to try their best on such tests. But older people just don't care much about nonsense words. What looks like a diminished ability in the elderly may partly be lack of interest."

Firmly convinced that conventional testing unjustly penalizes older people, Stephen W. Cornelius and Avshalom Caspi designed a more comprehensive intelligence-measuring instrument called the Everyday Problem-Solving Inventory (EPSI). Questions test practical intelligence (the ability to size up situations and determine appropriate strategies) as well as social competence (the ability to tolerate differences and effect compromises). Older volunteers consistently do better on the EPSI than younger volunteers. This may not prove that "older means wiser" across the board, but it does indicate that there are different, equally "smart" modes of intelligence and that old age can give just as much as it takes away.

Tragically, despite all the contradictory evidence, the belief persists that the older you get after sixty, the stupider you get, and this belief can easily turn into a self-fulfilling prophecy. Older people can, of course, succumb to senility, but senility is a disease that strikes a small percentage of older brains and is not a natural part of the aging process. Dr. Walter Shaie, an expert on aging, remarks, "Those who don't accept the stereotype of a helpless old age, but instead feel they can do as well in old age as they have at other times in their lives, don't become ineffective before their time."

The best way to ensure that you stay at the top of the class in your senior years is to stay mentally active. Read, write, and travel. Take courses. Pursue challenging hobbies. And above all, be sure to include young people as well as old people in your social life: Young dogs *can* learn old tricks.

Can Specific Foods or Drugs Enhance My Intelligence?

Throughout human history, various digestible commodities—appetizing or not—have been touted as brain foods. In Biblical times, the lowly lentil was so honored. Medieval European sages sought wisdom from more exotic fare, such as pulverized lizard or eagle hearts, while their Asian contemporaries sipped ginkgo tea for the same purpose. And at the very onset of the Age of Reason, the court of Louis XVI revived an ancient Greek practice and nibbled on gold leaf, hoping it might stimulate their gray matter.

Favorites have come and gone in rapid succession, but among all designated brain foods down through the ages, fish has been the most celebrated. As it turns out, modern medical authorities offer guarded support for this reputation. Fish is high in protein, and protein has been scientifically proven to be vital to the health and growth of neurons. Dr. Wayne Bidlack, associate professor at the

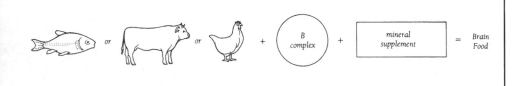

University of Southern California School of Medicine, remarks, "For centuries, people have thought that fish somehow helps develop the brain's capacity. However, a lot of that has to do with the simple fact that people who get their recommended daily allowance [RDA] of protein, along with all the other nutrients, will naturally tend to think more clearly and be more [mentally] active."

The RDA for protein is approximately forty-four grams for women and fifty-six grams for men. More than this amount, warns Bidlack, won't do the brain any good and may even be self-defeating, since the added protein will only be converted to waste matter. Two average servings of fish and two generous servings of dairy food per day will meet the RDA requirement, but, as far as the brain is concerned, you can replace the fish with red meat or chicken (or pulverized lizard or eagle hearts).

Recent studies have shown that vitamins and minerals are just as important to brain functioning as protein. In 1981, the National Academy of Science released the details of a study conducted by Dr. Ruth Harrell involving sixteen children classified as mentally retarded. After receiving a vitamin and mineral supplement for eight months, the subjects scored significantly higher on intelligence tests. Comparable results were achieved in a similar 1988 experiment conducted with ninety twelve- and thirteen-year-old British schoolchildren of average intelligence. At the end of eight months, those students who had been taking a vitamin and mineral supplement showed a remarkable increase in nonverbal intelligence scores compared to those students who had been taking a placebo. Explaining why the increase occurred only in nonverbal intelligence scores, one of the researchers stated, "Inadequate nutrition would be expected to show its earliest effects on the more biological intelligence measured by the nonverbal intelligence test. An increase in verbal intelligence might be expected only after the potential offered by a better nourished brain had been exploited by a stimulating environment."

B-complex vitamins play a particularly large role in proper neuron functioning. Vitamin B_{12}, for example, is crucially needed by the neuron to synthesize protein and fat. Because they eat no animal products (a major source of B-complex vitamins), vegetarians are at high risk for B_{12} deficiency, unless they make sure to tap such alternate sources as beans (including lentils!), sunflower seeds, peanuts, brown rice, asparagus, leafy greens, and broccoli.

The above-mentioned British experiment suggests that it is especially important to monitor our mineral intake if we want our brain to work as intelligently as it can. Prior to that experiment, all of the volunteers were meeting most of their RDA requirements for vitamins through their normal diet, but were satisfying only 50 percent or less of each mineral requirement. U.S. dietary studies show that this imbalance—adequate vitamin ingestion but subadequate mineral ingestion—is commonplace in America as well. Minerals like selenium, iron, zinc, iodine, chromium, molybdenum, boron, copper, and manganese are essential ingredients for optimum brain performance, and since it's difficult to ensure that our mineral needs will consistently be met by our daily diet (minerals are the first nutrients lost in food processing), a mineral supplement may be advisable.

Regrettably, no drugs currently on the market will compensate for a brain-debilitating diet or will make the smart eater even smarter. There is an experimental drug called nimodipine that appears to enable the brains of old rabbits to learn as well—or better—than the brains of young rabbits. Presumably, it does so by blocking neurons from absorbing excess calcium, which can impair brain functioning both in rabbits and humans (and which is not directly related to calcium levels in their diets). Researchers at Northwestern University have "every reason to believe" that nimodipine has widespread human applications, but for now, the Food and Drug Administration will only approve its use for victims of certain types of strokes.

Meanwhile, as you wait for more medical breakthroughs regarding brain foods and drugs, try drinking more ginkgo tea. According to recent research, *Ginkgo biloba* extract does seem to have a pharmacologic effect on the circulatory system, increasing the flow of nutrients and oxygen to the brain. You'd do well to hold back on your gold-leaf consumption, though. Remember: Louis XVI and most of his court lost their heads entirely.

"IDIOT" SAVANTS

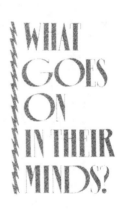

WHAT GOES ON IN THEIR MINDS?

Thanks to the Oscar-winning 1988 film *Rain Man,* millions of people now have a clear image to associate with that rare and baffling phenomenon, the "idiot" savant. Dustin Hoffman's character Raymond Babbitt can't perform the simplest addition or subtraction tasks, yet he knows at a glance the exact number of toothpicks that have spilled out of a full box. He is mentally incapable of making a phone call, but he can memorize an entire phone book at a single sitting. He is unable to take care of himself on a day-to-day basis; nevertheless, he easily racks up a fortune in Las Vegas, "outwitting" the dealers by keeping track of the cards.

Properly speaking, Raymond the Rain Man is a victim of savant syndrome—mentally and emotionally subcompetent except for a streak of astounding brilliance. In the century since the syndrome was first identified by J. Langdon Down (more famous as the articulator of Down's syndrome), its victims have been tagged "idiot" savants; but aside from being derogatory, the label is inaccurate. By definition, an "idiot" has an IQ lower than twenty-five. In actuality, most victims of savant syndrome possess an IQ of forty or more. Nor is the syndrome exclusive to the mentally retarded. In 20 percent of the 200 cases on record, it happened to people of normal intelligence as the result of a brain injury or a grave episode of mental illness.

The term "savant" (from the French *savoir,* "to know") does capture the victim's tendency to perform certain knowledge-related tasks with uncanny skill, but the range of potential abilities is always severely limited. Typically, the victim demonstrates a finite number of talents associated with musical expression, performance in the visual arts, mechanical construction, mathematical calculation, rote (word-for-word) memory, or eidetic (image-pattern) memory. Here are some examples of extraordinary cases.

- In Down's time, the Englishman James Henry Pullen was known as "the genius of Earlswood Asylum." He spent most of his life producing exquisite works of carpentry and drawing, with a special flair for ship design. Today, his two workshops are open to the public.
- Leslie Lemke, now thirty-six years old, gives virtuoso piano concerts despite being blind, palsied, and mildly retarded. After listening to an audience member play or sing a musical piece, familiar or not, Lemke can not only reproduce it perfectly (including any mistakes made by the challenger), but also run it through a set repertoire of different compositional arrangements.
- "John" and "Michael," twenty-six-year-old twin savants studied by the famous American neurologist Dr. Oliver Sacks in 1966, excelled in one of the oddest feats connected with savant syndrome. Given any calendar date—May 5, 1912 or Christmas 8668—they could instantly calculate the day of the week for that date, even taking leap years into account. They lost this ability (as many savants do) during later rehabilitation.

The screen character Raymond Babbit differs somewhat from his real-life models. For the sake of stronger cinematic impact, his movements are swifter and jerkier, his expression is more disturbingly robotic, and he succumbs more easily to being touched than the typical savant. He's true to form, however, in most key respects. Like many victims of savant syndrome, he focuses obsessively on details, creates strange, ritualistic approaches to daily life events, and shows no evidence of understanding symbolic meanings or the basic "how" and "why" of things. Indeed, Raymond is autistic, which means he is psychologically withdrawn to the point where it is difficult, if not impossible, for him to express thoughts and feelings or to interact productively with others.

Savant syndrome occurs more often among autistics than any other group. The obsessive concentration that so often accompanies autism seems to favor the development of savant syndrome, which features a similar brand of detachment and inner intensity. Speaking of autistic savants, Dr. Thomas Hurley, director of the Institute of Noetic Sciences, explains, "If you imagine attention being like a light, theirs is like a laser rather than a broad-spectrum beam." It is this laserlike attention that miraculously enables autistic savants to translate in an instant the number of toothpicks spilled on the floor, to engrave the phone book into their memory as they read it, or to race through an endlessly repetitive pattern of day names and day numbers to pinpoint the precise day of the week for a precise date.

The factors that cause savant syndrome to develop in the human brain are as difficult to trace as the effects are to explain. Experts now lean toward one or more of the following three theories.

It's a subconscious compensation mechanism. Because the victims cannot engage in abstract reasoning or imaginative daydreaming, they compulsively throw all their efforts into more trivial mental tasks involving concrete details and patterns.

It's the product of a hormonal malfunction that creates imbalances between the right brain and the left brain. As a result, certain functions (such as left-brain calculating activities or right-brain spatial-recognition activities) may evolve disproportionately to each other. In abnormally high levels, the male hormone testosterone can impair neuron development; therefore, some researchers speculate, an overabundance of testosterone in the early months of fetal life may lead to problems in the development of coordination between the right brain and the left brain, which in turn may lead to savant syndrome. This theory would also explain why the overwhelming majority of savant syndrome victims are male.

It's the outcome of a freak change in the way the brain handles its memory system. Instead of a given impression or piece of information being appropriately processed as a *semantic* memory (facts and concepts) or an *episodic* memory (autobiographical experience), it is inappropriately processed as a more primitive *skill* memory. (See page 69 for further discussion of these three types of memory.) Thus, the original impression or information is stripped of any distracting emotional or symbolic significance and, in some special cases, is more easily and clinically remembered and retrieved.

◆◆◆◆◆◆◆◆◆◆

For now, simply cataloging the wondrous activities performed by victims of savant syndrome opens windows onto the marvels of the human mind. In the future, understanding how the savant's mind works might enable each of us to streamline at will our capacity to absorb and transmit different kinds of knowledge.

How Can I Tap into My Brain's Creative Potential?

You don't have to be a successful artist, scientist, or social maverick to be a creative person. As a child, you led a very creative life. Your youthful brain explored, questioned, and interpreted the world in all sorts of exciting and magically empowering ways. Otherwise, you would never have evolved into a functional human being.

As a grown-up, your brain remains fully capable of the same type of imaginative approach to life; but to realize that potential, you need to shake your mind free from the routines and conventions of adult thinking that can so easily enslave it. Here are some expert guidelines.

Play. Throughout his career, Sir Alexander Fleming, the discoverer of penicillin, loved to "paint" pictures with living germs—a mother and child, a ballerina, his house.

The activity served as a welcome break from the strict discipline of scientific methodology and helped him to learn even more about the colors, textures, and growth rates of different microorganisms. "It is striking how many great scientists have incorporated play into their work," comments Robert S. Root-Bernstein, a psychologist at Michigan State University. "One mental quality that facilitates discovery is a willingness to goof around."

Practice different modes of expression. Don Campbell, author of *Introduction to the Musical Brain,* once had the daunting task of teaching the alphabet to learning disabled students. Since their minds were completely blocked when it came to writing the letters, Campbell had the children walk the letters, trace them with their elbows, and, finally, dance them in succession. To his amazement, all his pupils could recite the alphabet at the end of a single class.

"Certain ways of singing, chanting, moving, create dynamic changes in brain waves," Campbell says. "Using the whole body to learn opens the channels between mind and body. It activates in the mind the image of what the body is doing."

If you have trouble expressing yourself in words, try singing, dancing, or drawing what you want to say. If you have difficulty with golfing, painting, or waltzing, try talking or writing it out.

Challenge the rules. Look at the world around you and make demands. In 1943, Edwin Land took a snapshot of his baby daughter at the seashore. Disturbed by her plea "Why can't I see the picture now, Daddy?" Land first got the idea for the Polaroid camera. Ask yourself in what ways your thinking and your methods of operation are passive, conventional, predictable, or dogmatic. Consider trying "opposite" ways of thinking or operating, purely as a catalyst for inspiration.

Break habits. Routines in our life-style can lead to routines in our thinking patterns. Both kinds of routines can be efficient and comfortable, but they can also place limits on our creativity. Every now and then, we need to take risks and expose ourselves to novel circumstances for the sake of stimulating our imagination.

Both Sides Now

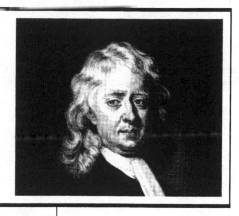

The English mathematician and natural philosopher Sir Isaac Newton (1642–1727) constantly experimented with different ways to expand his creative powers. He routinely spent hours and even days blindfolded to gain new sensory, emotional, and thinking perspectives. He also maintained a lifelong interest in alchemy, despite the fact that alchemical theory is so at odds with the basic principles of modern science that he helped articulate.

Sometimes just making the smallest shift in our behavior—even if it goes against our "better" nature—can work wonders. Jules Henri Poincaré, the famous French mathematician, once confessed, "For fifteen days I strove to prove that there could not be any functions like those I have since called Fuchsian functions. I was then very ignorant; every day I seated myself at my work table, stayed an hour or two, tried a great number of combinations and reached no results. One evening, contrary to my custom, I drank black coffee and could not sleep. Ideas rose in crowds; I felt them collide until pairs interlocked, so to speak, making a stable combination. By the next morning I had established the existence of a class of Fuchsian functions."

Turn accidents to your advantage. To our rational, habit-conditioned minds, an unfamiliar idea can seem frivolous, threatening, or impossible, when in fact it represents a stroke of genius. Similarly, an unanticipated event can initially be dismissed as an interruption, an aberration, or an accident, when it is actually an opportunity for a creative breakthrough. Had an apple not fallen by chance on Sir Isaac Newton's head, he may never have developed his revolutionary theory of gravity. If a factory worker had not inadvertently let a stirrer run overtime in a soap vat, Ivory Soap may never have floated.

As you go your scheduled way through life, remain alert for chances to capitalize on what fate unexpectedly brings you. The next time you have a sudden delay or detour in your travel plans, or you forget to bring home some work you were going to do, or a meteorite crashes into your vegetable garden, treat it as a creative challenge and make the most you can of it.

Brainware

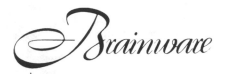

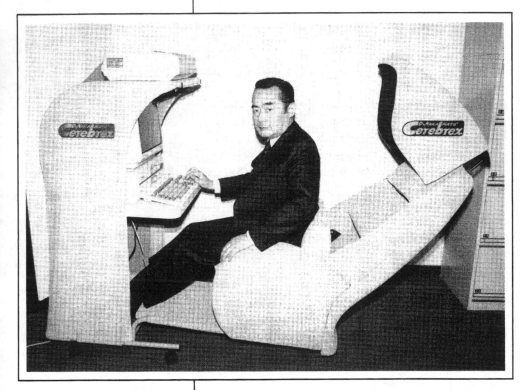

Cerebrex (and its inventor, Dr. Yoshiro NakaMats)

Cerebrex

Yoshiro NakaMats, often called the "Edison of Japan" because he holds the world record of 2,360 patents, has now brought us the Cerebrex, a chair-and-headset combo that sends sound waves into the user's head and feet. As the frequency gradually increases, NakaMats asserts, so does the flow of oxygen-carrying hemoglobin to the brain. The result is a sharp rise in intellectual prowess. Eighteen years in the making, the Cerebrex is very controversial, especially since NakaMats keeps promoting new and better benefits for users. He claims, for example, that it will put more zip in your sex life and even postpone aging. People who have availed themselves of the Cerebrex, however, insist that they emerge much more mentally acute, comparing the effect to a full night's sleep or a jolt of inspiration.

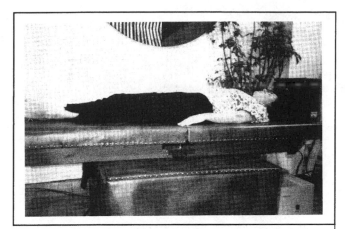

Graham Potentializer

The purpose of the Graham Potentializer is to boost one's "neuroefficiency" quotient and, by extension, one's intellectual performance by balancing the brain's natural electrical field. It works to accomplish this feat in two ways: by surrounding the user with its own electrical field, and by subjecting the user's body to a steady circular motion. You lie on a cot, and, while a small electronic box at your head emits its field, the cot smoothly and slowly rotates you clockwise and counterclockwise on the horizontal. The box's electrical field acts as a stabilizing environment in which the brain can realize its own personal best wavelengths, and the motion replicates the brain-awakening physical activities associated with childhood (a rhythmic agitation of the fluid in the inner ear reportedly stimulates neurons). With repeated use, brain cells allegedly grow stronger and develop more connective links.

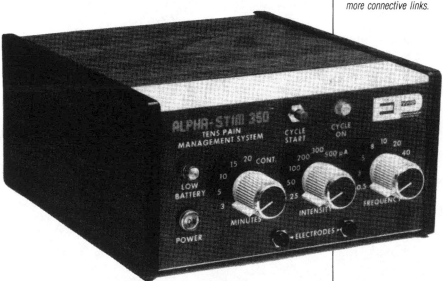

Alpha Stim

Combining electronic circuitry with computer technology, the Alpha-Stim is designed to provide tailor-made transcranial electrotherapy (TCET). The user directs an extremely low-amperage current through electrodes attached to a headband, and the resulting stimulation, according to Joseph Light of Biochemical Instruments Co. Inc., releases vasopressin and other mind-enhancing peptides. Devotees claim that by setting the Alpha-Stim to your proper waveform (which you quickly discover through practice), you will activate your brain's learning pathways and improve your ability to think. The enhancement lasts as long as you remain "hooked" and for several hours afterward.

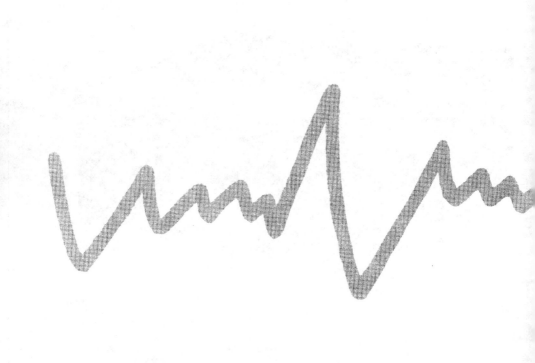

5

EMOTIONS

*O*ver two millennia after Aristotle first
identified the heart as the center of
emotions, we still tend to believe it.
We declare love to be "an affair of the heart";
if love fails, we're "heartbroken." The brain,
by contrast, is dubbed "the organ of intellect." In fact, the brain is just as responsible
for our emotional life as it is for our rational
life, and the two are inextricably related.

That the brain's limbic system has specific
mechanisms for generating emotions was first
proven in 1954 by scientists in Montreal,
who discovered that rats apparently feel intense pleasure when an electrical current is
directed through a particular region of the
hypothalamus (once trained to turn on that
current by pressing a lever, the rats would
press the lever incessantly). In subsequent ex-

periments, the same researchers provoked feelings of aversion in rats by stimulating another section of the hypothalamus. They went on to establish the existence of a "calmness–rage" center in the amygdala (directly above the hypothalamus) as well as an "excitement–depression" center in the nearby septum pellucidum.

All the evidence implies that human brains function the same way. Whether you're talking about rat brains or human brains, however, the story doesn't stop at this

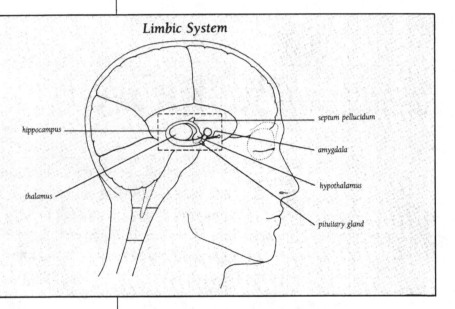

Limbic System

hippocampus

thalamus

septum pellucidum

amygdala

hypothalamus

pituitary gland

point. The limbic system may actually dispatch the neurochemicals that transmit specific emotional feelings, but it is not the sole emotion-producing agency. The cerebral cortex—the brain's data bank of personal experience—must first tell the limbic system what *quality* of response to make. Based on this electrochemical message, the limbic system regulates its reaction level from mild to extreme along the particular emotional spectrum that's been stimulated: pleasure–aversion, calmness–rage, excitement–depression. This close cooperation between the "thinking" cortex and the "feeling" limbic system means that each person (or rat) has a unique emotional life, depending on his or her own subjective background.

But can the whole world of human emotions be reduced to three general categories like pleasure–aversion, calmness–rage, and excitement–depression? Scientists claim that it can, though they bicker over terms. The vocabulary we use to describe our emotions is vast and complicated, they admit, but this is because emotions are so difficult to distinguish and interpret rationally. "Emotions tend to blend into each other, like colors,"

The Eyes Have It

Pupil size can be a fairly reliable indicator of a person's basic emotional state. (1) A small pupil indicates excitement or anger. (2) A pupil about twice as wide as the colored rim around it indicates peacefulness or sexual "openness"; in fact, people tend to find pupils of this size more attractive than smaller ones. (3) A very large pupil suggests fear, but if it's this large, it may indicate a complete lack of interest—the pupil owner is probably either asleep or almost comatose!

remarks Stanford University's Dr. Gordon Bower. "A few primary emotions can be mixed in various proportions to create other emotions. For example, sadness mixed with surprise may blend into disappointment." Sadness and surprise themselves may both be colors in the excitement–depression category; similarly, joy, hope, love, contentment, hate, grief, and fear may all be shades of the pleasure–aversion palette.

We can, however, get too carried away with the whole notion of sources and causes when it comes to describing the way in which the brain produces emotions. Like the intellectual process, the emotional process owes less to specific locations in the brain than it does to the intricate circuitry that connects all the different brain locations and determines the brain's overall, moment-by-moment response to life. A given emotional experience is heavily influenced by the simultaneous nature of our health, consciousness, memories, thoughts, and situational circumstances, not to mention our personal history of related emotional experiences.

As for the effects of different emotional experiences, they also vary widely, according to our total state of being at the time as well as our learned and built-in patterns of behavior. All human beings, for example, exhibit pupil dilation when they're excited: Among other things, it's a powerful sexual-interest signal. Some individuals also sweat more, fidget, and make exclamatory noises. Comparatively few individuals actually break into hives, develop gastric ulcers, stutter, or smash furniture; but if they do, the reason lies in the manner in which their particular physical makeup combines with their particular psychological makeup at that particular moment.

Sometimes the emotion-producing interplay between the cortex and the limbic system gets interrupted; consequently, the effect of a given emotion is rendered far more uncontrollable than it might otherwise be. Many strong psychotropic drugs, like cocaine, heroin, or phencyclidine (more commonly known as "PCP" or "angel dust") almost completely disengage the limbic system from the sobering mediation of the cortex, which typically results in violent mood swings and wildly impulsive physical actions. Drugs like alcohol and marijuana function the same way, but usually to a lesser degree. Similar problems are experienced by victims of episodic dyscontrol syndrome (EDS), whose occasional periods of erratic emotional reactions can be traced to a head trauma, stroke, tumor, or developmental defects in childhood.

You'll learn more about physical manifestations of emotions in Chapter 6. This chapter focuses on the emotions themselves. "One thing that goes to the heart of human beings," states Dr. Philip Johnson-Laird, a renowned psychologist at England's Cambridge University, "is the importance of an emotional life. We take great pleasure in having our emotions moved either by the real world or by imaginary events." The articles that follow are designed to help you make the best of your emotional life. They explore ways in which you can tame undesirable emotions, like despair and hostility, and enhance desirable emotions, like joy and love. They also assist you in dealing with such complex and widespread emotional problems as phobias, manic depression, and—last, but by no means least—seasonal funks.

How Can I Achieve Better Control Over My Emotions?

The word "emotion" itself, from the Latin e ("out") plus movere ("to move"), suggests the personal value we can derive from our emotions. They bestir us, so that we don't sink into a life of habit or inertia. They transport our imagination beyond the narrow confines of reason. They surprise us and keep us flexible to change. Certain "moving out" experiences, however, are too jarring to be beneficial in these ways. And for some individuals, "moving out" becomes a calamitous way of life—a never-ending roller coaster ride that makes it difficult to function productively. How can you avoid or manage specific emotional problems? What can you do to prevent your emotions from completely taking over your life? Here are some brain-work suggestions.

Study Your Emotional Life and Develop Self-Help Strategies. Our emotional reactions to a life situation is based on how we *perceive* it, so we need to monitor our perceptions carefully. Dr. Aaron T. Beck of the University of Pennsylvania explains, "If we see things as negative, we feel negative and behave in a negative way. If we see things as pleasant, we behave in a positive way and have positive feelings. As long as we perceive reality properly, it's good for us to be rewarded when things go well and punished when they go badly. The trouble arises when a person sees things negatively, but his perceptions are inaccurate."

When we're emotionally troubled, we tend to exaggerate or overgeneralize. "There's nothing I can do," we say. "It's hopeless. It's the worst thing that could happen." We're also inclined to take certain emotional upheavals too personally, and assume that we're somehow wrong or incompetent as human beings. In task-performance experiments with two groups of people—one emotionally stable, the other not—Beck found that the stable volunteers credited their successes to skill, their failures to bad luck. The unstable ones credited their successes to luck, their failures to lack of skill.

Finally, we can greatly aggravate our emotional difficulties by brooding on them in solitude. "People with psychological problems tend to spend more time alone and feel the worse for it," notes Dr. Reed Larson of the University of Illinois. "Bulimics [abnormally voracious eaters], for example, are fine when they are with other people but completely fall apart when they are alone."

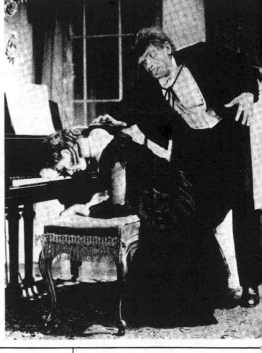

In Robert Louis Stevenson's short novel *Dr. Jekyll and Mr. Hyde*, the Mr. Hyde character represents the emotional beast that lurks inside even the most socially well-adjusted human being, as symbolized by Dr. Jekyll. The Victorian notion that civilization is based upon the control of one's emotions profoundly influenced Sigmund Freud.

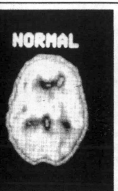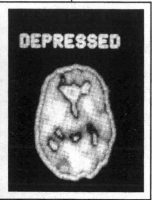

NORMAL DEPRESSED

On the left is a PET scan of a normal person. On the right is a PET scan of a depressed person. The sharp contrast between the two PET scans proves that depression can have organic roots. (See page 30 for more information on PET scans.)

While your basic emotional temperament may not change much during your lifetime, you can make signficant day-to-day adjustments in the way you perceive events and respond to them. When you face an emotionally trying situation, guard against exaggerating or over-generalizing, and focus instead on your specific options for taking direct action. Avoid putting yourself down by doing something that will exercise your good traits. And seek the company of others, whether it's to gather more rational views on the situation or simply to change your mood.

Check Possible Physical Causes for Your Emotional Problems. Many ills of the body can have an insidious effect on the mind, even before they produce other, more tangible symptoms. Most pervasive among those physical maladies that can affect your brain chemistry—and, therefore, your emotional life—are blood-sugar irregularities (which may lead to hypoglycemia, hyperglycemia, or diabetes), high or low blood pressure, and allergies. Far less common physical sources of emotional disturbances are brain lesions and tumors. Describe any troubling emotional patterns to your physician and seek advice regarding possible physical explanations and appropriate testing and treatment procedures. Your physician can also tell you whether you're experiencing bad emotional side effects from medications you're taking.

You can also be your own doctor and try to determine whether there's any connection between your emotional problems and your use of alcohol, recreational drugs, or steroids (which can have devastating effects on your blood chemistry). You may drink, smoke, swallow, snort, or shoot-up almost daily just to feel good or perform well, unaware that you're setting up a dangerous cycle of emotional dependency. Or an underlying anxiety or depression may be driving you to toxic substance abuse, in which case you are denying a serious problem instead of dealing with it. Recent studies conducted by Dr. Janusz Rybakowski of the Polish Medical Academy intimate that

132

as many as three out of four alcoholics may drink to overcome alexithymia, an inability to feel or express emotions easily.

Consider Getting Professional Help. If an emotional problem is too strong for you to handle on your own, enlist qualified guidance. There are many different types of therapists, from mental health counselors (bachelor's degree, possible master's degree, plus job training), to psychologists (PhD), to psychiatrists (MD). There are also many different types of therapies. Some are named after their founders, such as Freudian or Jungian psychoanalysis (for more information on Freudian and Jungian psychoanalysis, see Chapter 2). Others are named after their procedures, such as gestalt therapy, which involves coaxing the client to reenact emotionally challenging experiences. Whether they are single-day, six-week, or six-year endeavors, all such therapies can involve any combination of these three approaches: (1) *cognitive,* one-to-one dialogue between a client and a therapist aimed at correcting problems in the client's perceptions; (2) *behavioral,* one-to-one dialogue and role-playing between a client and a therapist aimed at correcting problems in the client's daily feelings and self-management; (3) *interpersonal,* dialogue and role-playing among a group of clients and a therapist aimed at correcting problems in the clients' social and communication skills.

> *Most people are about as happy as they make up their minds to be.*
> —Abraham Lincoln

It is important to shop around before determining which therapist and therapy seem most suited to you. Do some research at the library. Talk with friends and relatives who have had therapy. Request information from your local public health service and relevant state or national organizations (such as the American Psychological Association and the American Psychiatric Association, both in Washington, D.C.). And confer with several potential therapists before making a final decision. The therapist you choose should be someone you trust who has similar ideas about what form your treatment should take.

MANIC-DEPRESSIVES

WHAT GOES ON IN THEIR MINDS?

Like the weather, Roger's life is a difficult-to-predict succession of highs and lows. When he's high, he's bursting with energy. He thinks fast, speaks fast, and acts fast, sometimes so fast that he can't keep up with himself. Deliriously convinced of his God-given right and power to do anything he wants, he'll spin grandiose plans for the future, go on extravagant shopping sprees, phone distant acquaintances in the middle of the night, and seek legal action against anyone who crosses him, no matter how slightly. When he's low, the exhilarating energy plummets. He moves slowly and exhibits delayed reactions, especially in conversation. Because he can't clearly remember his past actions, he's overcome with embarrassment, guilt, and paranoia. Anxious to escape from life, he sleeps longer and more deeply.

To his friends, Roger is an "interesting character." They never know whether he's going to be the life of the party, a charity case, or a pain in the neck. To his family, Roger is a wondrous force of nature—part superman, part madman. To science, Roger is a victim of bipolar disorder or, as it's more commonly known, manic depression. In essence, manic depression is an exaggerated form of the human condition, with its cycles of elation and despondency. As such, it can be very difficult to detect until it reaches an advanced stage, when the victim suffers extensive memory loss, bizarre delusions, and even hallucinations (technically symptoms of true mania, as opposed to "hypomania," the correct term for the high phase of manic depression).

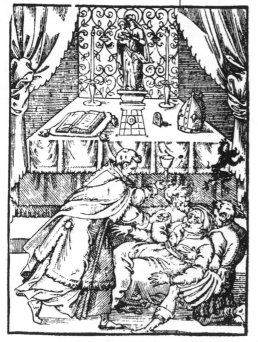

For most of human history, bipolar disorder and other forms of mental illness were unfairly associated with sin or evil. Here is a sixteenth-century depiction of an exorcism, in which a demon is seen leaving the body of a "possessed"—and, therefore, irrational—woman.

Aretaeus, the second-century Greek physician, first defined manic depression in the course of making his revolutionary distinction between *exogenous,* or externally caused, emotion (like anger at an uncooperative spouse) and *endogenous,* or internally caused, emotion (like a general sensation of anger without any outside explanation). He assumed the source of manic depression was "psychical," as did physicians throughout the Middle Ages, who blamed it on diabolical possession. Only in the twentieth century has manic depression been recognized as a chemical malfunction in the brain. Most scientists blame the disorder on irregularities in the brain's production of the neurotransmitter norepinephrine: Too much results in hypomania; too little, in depression. On a PET scan of a manic-depressive's brain, the disorder shows up as a distinctive light and dark pattern, indicating abnormalities in the brain's glucose consumption (an effect of the chemical imbalance that also causes bipolar disorder). High or low periods can last for hours, days, or weeks and take similar amounts of time to fluctuate.

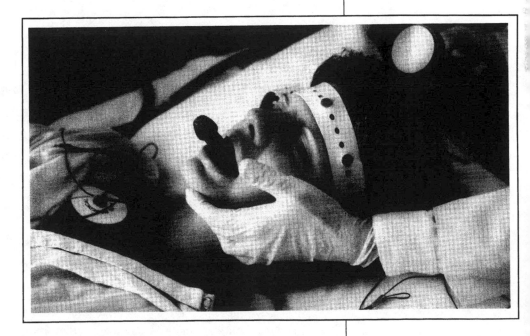

Electroshock therapy is sometimes the only potentially helpful treatment for people suffering from extreme cases of bipolar disorder. Contrary to popular belief, properly administered electroshock therapy does not create brain damage, nor does it cause any other negative aftereffects.

Treatment for manic depression varies according to the disorder's severity. Mild cases can usually be managed with ongoing medication. Lithium carbonate, which helps prevent extremes in the production of norepinephrine, is a common prescription. In strong cases, victims must often resort to electroconvulsive therapy: Low-grade electric current lasting for about a second is passed between electrodes attached to the scalp, causing a controlled seizure that disrupts manic-depressive electrochemical activity.

Regrettably, science cannot tell us how widespread manic depression is or how likely an individual is to develop it. Known cases account for a mere 1 percent of the American population, but experts estimate that this figure represents less than 10 percent of the actual victims, who either don't realize their troubling behavior has an organic cause or refuse to seek help out of denial, shame, or sheer orneriness. For some unknown reason, people of above-average education and/or affluence appear to be more at risk. And now science is in the process of proving what has long been suspected, that manic-depressive tendencies can be inherited.

In April 1987, Dr. Janice A. Egeland of the University of Miami released the results of a fascinating ten-year study on manic depression that she conducted among 12,000 Amish people in Lancaster County, Pennsylvania. Because the Amish community has historically been so tightly knit and has kept such detailed genealogical records, Egeland found it an ideal subject pool for her efforts to trace symptoms of manic depression from one generation to another. When individual reminiscences led her to suspect a particular bloodline of manic-depressives, she examined the chromosomes of living descendants and discovered a distinct genetic marker. While scientists unanimously agree that an active case of manic depression issues from multiple factors, Egeland's work suggests that people who bear this genetic marker have a 60 to 80 percent chance of eventually developing the disorder.

As tragic as manic depression can become to its victims and their loved ones, its high phase can occasionally lead to exceptional achievements. Although the incidence rate of manic depression among famous creative people is no greater than the incidence rate among the general population, there's little doubt that sustained bouts of hypomanic energy contributed to the work of many recognizably manic-depressive artists, like the painter Vincent Van Gogh and the poets Robert Lowell and John Berryman. In acknowledgment of this fact, the National Symphony Orchestra performed a special concert on October 30, 1988, at Washington, D.C.'s Kennedy Center, in conjunction with a National Institute of Mental Health symposium on manic depression. The program consisted entirely of music composed by scientifically identifiable manic-depressives, including Berlioz, Tchaikowsky, Handel, and Schumann. Unsympathetic critics might argue that a steady diet of such music could turn any hapless listener into a manic-depressive. Luckily, it takes much more than outside influences!

What Role Does My Brain Play in My Sex Life?

"You could say that love is a brain bath of dopamine and norepinephrine," declares Dr. Michael R. Liebowitz of Columbia University in New York City. For those of us who wouldn't know what we were saying, he translates: "Love depends on powerful perturbations of our normal brain chemistry." When we come into contact with a person who fits our notion of attractiveness, our production of the chemical neurotransmitters dopamine and norepinephrine shoots up, and this activates the "pleasure chest" in our brain's limbic system. But what accounts for our initial attraction? Is it something we decide for ourselves, or is our brain predisposed to make certain choices?

Scientists tell us that whatever kind of individual we personally come to consider "our type," we are all programmed from birth to favor the same basic attributes, according to our gender and sexual orientation. The human brain has evolved slowly over millennia in response to specific challenges that have persisted in its outside environment, so it makes sense that "natural selection" has left modern men and women with certain innate predispositions. An extensive study made by Dr. David Bass, a psychologist at the University of Michigan, reveals that women tend to be more attracted than men to a mate whose physical qualities suggest ambition and social success. The reason, Bass theorizes, stems from a woman's age-old need to avoid squandering her limited supply of eggs on a possible underachiever. By contrast, men, who remain (potentially) ever ready to supply sperm, place a higher value on physical qualities in a mate that suggest fertility.

This species pattern aside, we can and do develop other sexual cravings—complementary, contradictory, or totally unrelated. Some are taught to us by the culture in which

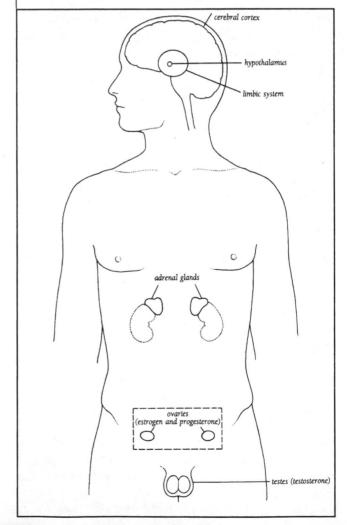

we mature. People in many impoverished or famine-prone societies, for example, especially prize fat people. Other sexual desires emerge from our own individual life histories, such as the attraction to a particular kind of smile, voice, walk, or personality trait.

However much our cerebral cortex, the locus of our "intellectual" mind, influences what does or does not stimulate our limbic system, the nature of our sexual response to such stimulation is still subject to inborn brain/body behavior patterns. Scientists currently speculate that the hypothalamus sets the sex hormones in motion. The most important of these hormones, for both men and women, is the male sex hormone testosterone (the female sex hormones estrogen and progesterone are important in ovulation and pregnancy, but play no role in the sex drive itself). Testosterone is released in the testes of men and in the adrenal glands of both men and women. Since the testes produce far more testosterone than the adrenal glands, men have roughly twenty times the amount that women have; but there is no direct relationship between testosterone levels and the intensity of one's sex drive, which is largely a psychological matter.

Once in motion, the sex drive follows an unvarying sequence, which experts divide into four phases. The first phase is *excitation:* The physical body undergoes the dilations and constrictions of blood vessels, organs, and tissues that prepare it for optimum sexual activity, in harmony with an emotional arousal governed by the limbic system. Next comes the *plateau* phase, when the body has achieved maximum readiness for sexual activity. The third phase is *orgasm,* the releasing of body fluids associated with sex, followed by the fourth and final *resolution* phase, which involves prolonged physical and emotional relaxation.

Thus we have the complete cycle of the sex drive, but not the whole trip about sex. As any long-term couple can testify, there's a distinct difference between "sexual attraction," which can occur with a stranger, and "sexual attachment," which can only be attained through increasing emotional involvement with the same individual. While "attraction" relationships may be more passionate, "attachment" relationships are, as a rule, more emotionally rewarding.

According to Liebowitz, both types of sexual love—attraction and atttachment—are "evolutionarily desirable," and, therefore, likely to be genetically built-in parts of our brain's repertoire of behaviors. Liebowitz also believes that attachment love, associated with a general reduction of anxiety and depression, may cause ongoing, beneficial chemical alterations in an area of the brain stem known as the *locus coeruleus,* which functions as an alarm center for such negative feelings.

One thing Liebowitz definitely does *not* believe is that sex as the brain expert knows it corresponds to sex as the lover knows it. For the lover, sex is inseparable from the whole multiemotional phenomenon commonly called "love." "The importance of love has nothing to do with brain chemistry," Liebowitz insists. "It has to do with the depth and variety of the pleasures experienced. Love is an opportunity for learning and a way to enhance our lives."

APHRODISIACS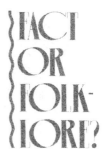

Aphrodite, the Greek goddess of love (worshipped as Venus by the Romans), is famous for her laugh. In classical verse, it beguiles the sternest misanthropes, taunts lovesick conquerors, and renders even the most brilliant thinkers tongue-tied and witless. How she must howl, then, over the sheer number of digestibles, named in her honor, that allegedly have the power to stimulate feelings of love and sensuality in the mortal brain.

Because Aphrodite is said to have sprung full-grown from the sea (*aphros* being Greek for "foam"), it seems at least mythologically logical that so many supposed aphrodisiacs also have a marine origin. Caviar, for example, has held a strong, unbroken reputation as an aphrodisiac since the time of Homer. Not only do fish eggs come from the sea, but they also occupy a key position in the reproductive cycle. Nevertheless, the case for caviar as an aphrodisiac rests entirely on circumstantial evidence. As a relatively rare and expensive commodity, caviar is associated with special occasions, lending it a seductive element of glamour, and its salty taste encourages wine-drinking, which, in turn, lowers one's inhibitions. As an organic compound, caviar has no more ability to trigger affection or lust than beer nuts or cocktail weenies.

It's the same fishy story with other seaborn aphrodisiacs of popular acclaim. Tom Jones, the title character of Henry Fielding's famous eighteenth-century English novel, is reportedly turned on by lobster, but there's no dietary support for this theory. In his memoirs, Casanova swears by oysters, calling them "a spur to the spirit and to love," but consider the source—a stud who needed very little spurring. Clams, too, are falsely lauded as passionate fare ("Venus on the half-shell" notwithstanding).

Many experts speculate that seafood appears to have aphrodisiac properties because it is rich in phosphorus, a bladder excitant. A similar kind of reputation by association may also play a part in the appeal of clams and oysters to the would-be lover—their physical structure suggests the female sex organ. So does the structure of a peach, with its fuzzy cleft. Peaches were especially prized as aphrodisiacs in eighteenth- and nineteenth-century Europe, where they were novel delicacies. A "peach house" became English slang for a house of prostitution, and a sexually alluring young woman was (and still is) called a "peach" in virtually every European language. The physical structure of the male sex organ has also inspired its fair share of aphrodisiac designations. Witness the cult of the rhinoceros horn (which is powdered for consumption), the pickle, the mushroom, or the mandrake root, (which figures in many root-based recipes for the notorious—and "groundless"—love potion, Spanish Fly).

Finally, there are the candy aphrodisiacs, and here science does have disarming news for Venus. The high carbohydrate content of chocolate and honey in particular steeply escalates the brain's production of serotonin, a neurotransmitter that generates warm, mellow feelings. Even more to the point, recent, highly sophisticated analyses of chocolate have revealed small amounts of phenylethylamine, a chemical naturally produced in the brain that many researchers believe increases when a person experiences erotic attraction. In short, eating bonbons on Valentine's Day may, indeed, put you in the mood for love.

What Causes Phobias, and How Can They Be Cured?

Chances are you have a phobia, but that doesn't mean you're a basically fearful person, or that you have a mental disorder, or that you risk going crazy or dying of fright. Despite its ominous-sounding Latin tag, a phobia is nothing more than an "ongoing and unreasonable fear of something." The American Psychiatric Association tells us that over 16 million people in the United States actually profess their phobic nature, but very few nonprofessing Americans can claim that they're completely free of an ongoing and unreasonable fear of something.

For the sake of diagnostic convenience, phobias are divided into four categories: (1) animal phobias; (2) social phobias (fear of doing something in public); (3) agoraphobia (fear of the outside world, from the Greek word *agora* or "marketplace"); and (4) specific phobias. This last category, by far the most prevalent, refers to fears that center around one particular object or situation. Among the most common specific phobias are acrophobia (fear of heights), claustrophobia (fear of enclosed spaces), and hydrophobia (fear of water). But the list extends to such items as:

Algophobia–fear of pain

Arachibutyrophobia–fear of getting peanut butter stuck to the roof of your mouth

Astraphobia–fear of storms, lightning, thunder

Belonephobia–fear of pins, needles, injections

Decidophobia–fear of decisions

Ergophobia–fear of work

Gephydrophobia–fear of crossing bridges

Hematophobia–fear of blood

Iatrophobia–fear of doctors

Logizomechanophobia–fear of computers or computing

Monophobia–fear of being alone

Nosophobia–fear of disease

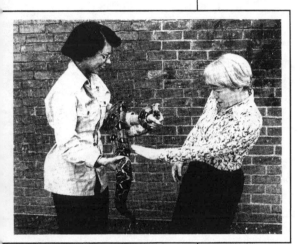

The fear of snakes, or herpetophobia, is one of the most common animal phobias, as reflected throughout human cultural history—from stories of Eve and the serpent, Hercules and the Hydra, and Saint George and the dragon, to customs like snake-handling as a courageous act of faith among Christian fundamentalists.

Nucleomitiphobia—fear of a nuclear bomb explosion
Phobophobia—fear of one's own fears
Pyrophobia—fear of fire
Sophophobia—fear of learning
Taphephobia—fear of being buried alive
Technophobia—fear of technology
Thanatophobia—fear of death
Vestiphobia—fear of wearing clothes

According to Dr. Leslie Solyom of Montreal's McGill University, most phobias develop when some traumatic life event rekindles an unpleasant experience from early childhood. The catalytic life event may be unrelated to the phobia itself. For example, a four-year-old boy on his first day of school may suffer a strong anxiety that his subconscious mysteriously relates to an infant memory of being frightened by a housefly. The result could be the genesis of entomophobia, the fear of insects. The first day of school and the long-ago day he was frightened by an insect may have nothing at all in common except perhaps for a certain type or degree of fear. A twenty-one-year-old woman experiencing intense pressure at work may subconsciously connect that "entrapped" feeling to a grade school memory of being cornered by an unknown assailant, which could engender xenophobia, the fear of strangers. Fundamentally, a phobia is the mind's way of handling "diffuse" or unexpressible anxiety: Memory gives this fear a focal point, and an unusually fixated pattern of stimulus-and-response concerning that focal point develops between the brain's limbic system and frontal lobes.

Animal phobias tend to crystallize at a relatively young age. Social phobias and specific phobias can be acquired at any age, but typically the victim is an otherwise "reasonable" teenager. Victims of agoraphobia—the least focused and, in many ways, the most crippling phobia—tend to be in their midtwenties or older, an age when world-weariness can reach fearsome proportions.

Popular wisdom says, "Live with your phobia. You'll get over it eventually." In practice, this is not good advice. The only

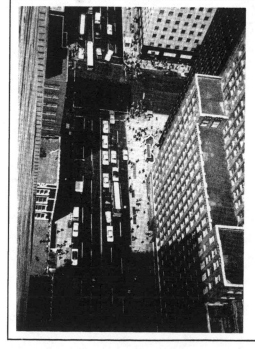

What's your response to this picture? Acrophobia, or fear of heights, is a widespread "specific phobia."

way to get rid of a phobia is to go through some deliberate process of desensitization. Behavioral therapists can disperse most phobias over time by leading the victim through imaginative exercises. At first, the victim is directed to envision the gentlest possible encounter with the object of his or her fear. Gradually, the confrontational scenarios are escalated in intensity, and, as the victim spends more and more time mentally coping with the focal point of the phobia, it hopefully loses its power to terrify. If behavorial therapy doesn't work, a combination of suggestion and drugs may be effective. After the phobia is deliberately invoked through guided visualization, the victim is injected with a relaxing sedative, such as phenelzine or any one of a number of barbiturate anesthetics. This may break the brain's phobic stimulus-response pattern.

In situations where the phobia is relatively mild, professional intervention is often unnecessary. Instead, the victim develops his or her own successful phobia-busting program. The following story comes from a woman who took it upon herself to conquer her agoraphobia.

> *O* *never hit*
> *a shot, not even in practice, without having a very sharp, in-focus picture of it in my head.*
> —Jack Nicklaus

> *I had to practice **staying** somewhere instead of running home in fear; so I'd park my car a block away and pull out my knitting. Knitting, because it is rhythmic, soothing, and creative, was just the diversion I needed to distract me from my self-defeating panic at being away from home. It was a **positive** action and, while it took many sessions of knitting in the car or some other "new" place for me to recover, I now drive to and from a full-time job—still with my knitting, but not as a crutch. I simply enjoy doing it [from* No Idle Hands: The Social History of American Knitting *by Anne L. MacDonald, New York: Ballantine, 1988].*

SEASONAL AFFECTIVE DISORDER

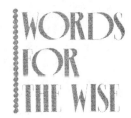
WORDS FOR THE WISE

December rolls around, and 'tis the season to be jolly, right? 'Tis not, brain experts say, for possibly up to one-third of the total U.S. population, whose winter is destined to be gloomy rather than joyful. In extreme cases, this gloom manifests itself as deep depression, accompanied by lethargy, an inability to concentrate, and bouts of a strong craving for carbohydrates—all symptoms of a syndrome known as seasonal affective disorder or, appropriately, SAD.

SAD is directly tied to seasonal changes in natural light, as registered on the retina and processed in the brain. In winter, as we experience more hours of darkness each day, the brain directs its pineal gland to secrete greater amounts of the hormone melatonin, which tends to decrease our alertness and make us sleepier. Most of us barely notice the change, but others react more strongly. Why certain people develop full-blown SAD and others don't is not yet known. It's assumed that a combination of physiological and psychological factors are involved, similar to those connected with such behavioral disorders as carbohydrate-craving obesity syndrome (COS) and premenstrual syndrome (PMS). But geography also plays a role. Because winter hours of daylight are fewer in higher latitudes, the odds that you'll fall victim to SAD are about 1 in 1,000 if you live in the northern half of the United States, compared to about 1 out of 16,000 if you live in the southern half. Also, you're more likely to succumb to SAD if you spend most of each winter day inside.

Once the source of SAD was established, it wasn't too difficult for science to find a cure. Victims almost always recover within less than a week if they institute a program of regular exposure to banks of high-intensity light: specifically, at least forty-five minutes each morning in front of full-spectrum lamps. A midwinter escape to the tropics works even faster, but the effects don't survive the return trip.

While winter's SAD tale may be the bleakest time-and-mood story of the year, the other seasons bring their own characteristic emotional turbulence. "For some people, April is indeed the cruelest month," notes the National Institute of Mental Health's Dr. Norman E. Rosenthal, quoting T. S. Eliot's poem *The Waste Land.* Suicides and hospital admissions for depression and alcoholism, Rosenthal states, reach an annual high in early spring. Why this happens he isn't sure, but the answer may lie in the infamous "spring fever" we all tend to feel at that time of year—a restlessness attributable to the increasing brilliance and longevity of daylight, which sharply reduces our melatonin level.

Come summer, certain unfortunate people experience an excess of anxiety that translates into long periods of acute despair interspersed with frequent panic attacks. Some authorities assume that this emotional state is the manic counterpart to SAD. They treat it with cooling face masks, which not only diminish the victim's exposure to natural light but also lower the temperature of blood circulating through his or her brain. Often, however, this therapy doesn't work. Dr. Thomas Wehr, a colleague of Rosenthal, believes that such bad cases of the summertime blues may stem from disorders in a latent hibernation pattern (aestivation, or summer hibernation, is a brain-driven energy-management system that activates in many animals when it's hot and dry). By contrast, Princeton University's Dr. Peter Mueller thinks that excessive anxiety in the summer may signal an organic mental illness, which he's labeled "seasonal energy syndrome (SES)." Lately, Muel-

In a recent study conducted by Michael Terman of the New York State Psychiatric Institute, SAD victims in northern areas of the United States showed much more dramatic mood fluctuations from season to season than their "normal" counterparts.

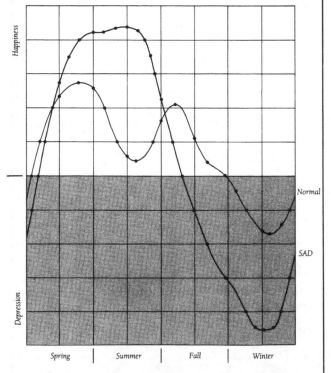

Happiness / Depression

Normal

SAD

Spring | Summer | Fall | Winter

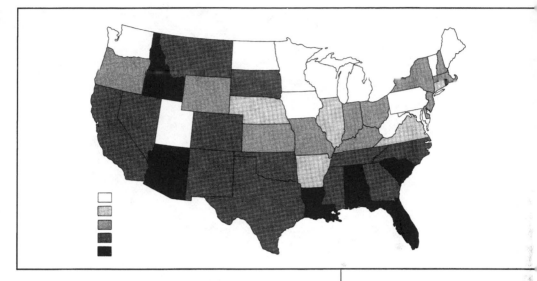

Based on data collated by researchers at the University of California (Irvine), this map indicates the relative percentage of people affected by SAD in each state of the continental United States. In Minnesota, the northernmost state, SAD claims over 100 people out of 1,000; in Florida, the southernmost state, it claims less than six people out of 100,000.

ler's theory is gaining credence due to experiments in which seizure-control drugs, normally prescribed to epileptics, are proving effective on so-called SES sufferers.

Assuming you successfully avoid SAD, spring fever, and SES, you may still be autumn's fall guy. Among the newest maladies recognized by psychiatrists these days is "post-vacation dysphoria," which is especially prevalent after Labor Day. During the summer, you're likely to experience more breaks from day-to-day stress as you spend more time enjoying the out-of-doors or taking recreational trips. When summer is over, the pain of resuming a more rigid schedule in a world that suddenly appears much more mundane can be quite upsetting. Many people cope by loading their calendars with social engagements, cultural activities, or sessions at the gym. Others initiate major life changes, seeking a new job, a new home, or a new image. And some turn immediately to their travel agent. "No question, we get a fair amount of people who, shortly after they get back from a summer vacation, visit us and make plans for their next trip," comments Wayne Berens, president of Revere Travel in Ewing, New Jersey. "Some people always have to have something on the fire."

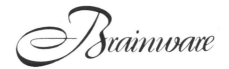

Brainware

Ionizer

Have you ever been exhilarated on a mountaintop, or depressed on a city street? Aesthetically speaking, it seems obvious that the former environment would be more conducive of enjoyment than the latter. One thing you may not realize, however—it is also more conducive atmospherically speaking. Mountain air, like the air at waterfalls or the seashore, consists of a healthy balance of positively and negatively charged atomic particles called ions. Where humans congregate to live and work, negative ions are destroyed by fumes, smoke, and dust outdoors and by heating and cooling systems indoors. What's left is electrified air, which can adversely change the chemical composition of neurotransmitters. We may wind up getting crabbier, more anxious, or more despondent than our situation warrants. Ionizers are brain fresheners, designed to increase the content of negative ions in the air and improve one's emotional well-being. Models come in a wide variety of sizes, from small units for automobiles to large floor models for hospital waiting rooms, auditoriums, and open-plan offices (places where ionizers are especially popular).

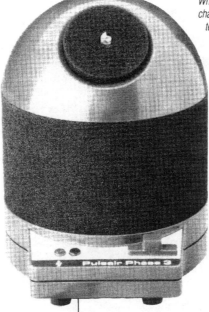

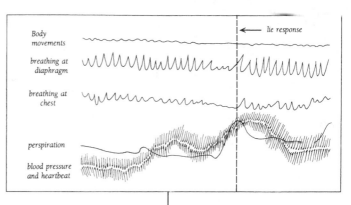

Body movements	
breathing at diaphragm	
breathing at chest	
perspiration	
blood pressure and heartbeat	

← lie response

Polygraph

We know it better as a lie detector, but a polygraph also helps to diagnose emotional problems. Attached to the user by electrodes and wires, a polygraph monitors how certain brain-regulated body movements fluctuate in response to questions or other investigatory stimuli, including inkblots, photographs, word association tests, or readings. A typical printout will display continuous line-drawing records of the user's breathing (at the diaphragm and the chest), perspiration, blood pressure, pulse, and galvanic skin response. Fluctuations in any or all of these line drawings indicate reactions fraught with emotional conflict. Lying is one such conflict, and so is concealing desire, suppressing anger, or denying fear. In a criminal case or the hiring of personnel, a polygraph can establish whether the user is knowingly guilty of not telling the truth about a real-life situation. In the context of psychological therapy, a polygraph can point to "unknown" as well as untold truths about the user's emotional life.

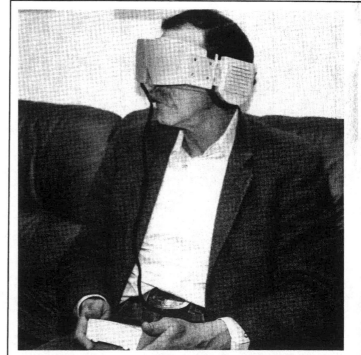

Tranquilite

As a quick, convenient antidote for depression and anxiety, the Tranquilite is one of the most effective machines in the New Age brain/mind arsenal. It consists of three interconnected and easily portable parts: thick, opaque goggles (fortunately lightweight); headphones; and a pocket-sized cartridge. The interior of the goggles is suffused by light, filling the wearer's field of vision with a blank, blue radiance. Meanwhile, the cartridge transmits soft, bubbling sounds through the earphones. The result is a lowering of blood pressure, heartbeat rate, and brain-wave frequency, and a cut in the production of mind-tensing biochemicals like adrenaline and cortisol—all of which makes the user feel relaxed, receptive, and renewed. The Tranquilite rarely spawns the kinds of altered states of consciousness one can experience inside an isolation tank (see page 64), but it works very well to restore the user's emotional equilibrium, especially if he or she is going through a period of intensified emotional reactions.

6

THE MIND-BODY CONNECTION

everal years ago, a man attended one
of Joseph Chilton Pearce's popular
child-raising seminars for the sole
purpose of comprehending an event that had
totally unnerved him. He had been at home
watching his eight-year-old son whittle. Suddenly the knife slipped and severed the arteries in his son's left wrist. As if in a trance,
the distraught father grabbed his son and
said, "Let's stop that blood!" Together, he
and his son stared at the gushing arteries and
shouted, "Blood, you stop that!" The bleeding

ceased. And in an abnormally short time, the wound healed.

Pearce's explanation came from years of studying children and unusual psychic phenomena: "He [the father] did not understand that the child is biologically geared to take reality cues from the parent; he did not know of the high suggestibility of the eight-year-old—or that [children of that age are] peculiarly susceptible to ideas about physical survival. But some part of him *did* know and broke through in the moment of emergency. All the son needed, of course, was the suggestion and the support."

Tales of mind over matter abound in the annals of parapsychology: mothers lifting cars that have rolled on top of their children; blind people regaining their sight in the ecstasy of good news; disembodied spirits of patients under surgery mentally choosing whether to live or to die. In certain contexts, this type of mind power can be deliberately engineered. Worshippers of voodoo, who invoke possession by spiritual entities known as loas, can withstand extreme exertion or fatigue and can even "outwit" deathly poisons. And at PK (for "psychokinesis") parties, amateur experimenters are able to walk across hot coals in their bare feet or bend silverware without moving a muscle.

From a scientific point of view, none of this evidence pointing to a strong, manipulable mind-body connection is valid. It doesn't conform to "typical" experience, and it can't be replicated using strict scientific methodology. Nevertheless, scientists do recognize that the mind and the body are interrelated in all sorts of ways that we can't yet articulate or control. Miraculous happenings aside, it's impossible to refute that everyday stress on the mind has an observable impact on the health of the body. Or that attacks of such diverse physical maladies as allergies, asthma, warts, ulcers, acne, canker sores, herpes, psoriasis, and lupus often conform precisely to the particular victim's mental and emotional crises. Or that chronic mind-related problems can lead to ongoing physi-

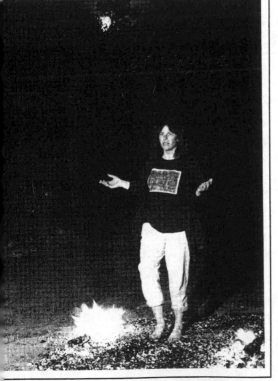

Call it "mob psychology" or "group pressure," it seems to facilitate such mind-over-matter stunts as fire-walking. So does the individual's own belief system.

cal malfunctions like stuttering, facial tics, impotence, frigidity, indigestion, constipation, high blood pressure, or insomnia.

In an effort to pin down more precisely how the body and the mind influence each other, scientists are busy finding new ways to employ the two main research strategies in their arsenal: field study and laboratory experiment. Their work in the field has been necessarily lengthy and painstaking. It involves charting the health histories of different personality types over extensive time periods, or following the lifelong careers of nonmedical healers, or exploring an entire human culture or subculture in depth. As for laboratory work, the potential scope of inquiry is severely limited from the start. A human being's mental and physical state of being is inextricably bound to real-life situations that are difficult, if not impossible, to re-create in an artificial environment. Ethical considerations also impose restrictions: There's a moral limit to how much stress you can deliberately impose on a subject, or how much you can jeopardize his or her physical well-being.

Despite these impediments to laboratory research, many substantial discoveries have been made in recent years. Some of these findings point to major breakthroughs in serious human health issues, like establishing how particular behaviors or states of mind aggravate or ameliorate life-threatening illnesses. Other findings are less monu-

The Magic Loop

Biofeedback machines, by means of which users can monitor and even affect their own body signals, have led to a revolution in mind-body therapy over the last two decades. Pictured here is Twilight Learning System's Model TL-1. Programmed to operate in response to the user's particular brain-wave state, it can serve a number of purposes, from inducing relaxation to enhancing one's retention of tape-recorded information.

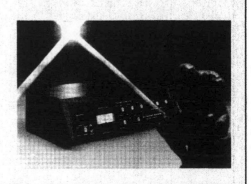

mental but still provocative. For instance, a 1988 study offers distressing proof that it is possible merely to look at food and gain weight. Time after time, when hungry, meat-loving subjects were exposed to a sizzling steak, their brains not only ordered an increase in saliva, but also upped insulin production, which automatically makes body cells store more fat. (However, weight gains from looking at food are, thank goodness, indeterminately small!)

For now, the most promising way in which medical science can intervene to exploit the mind-body connection is through the use of sophisticated electronic equipment known as biofeedback machinery. Sensors are hooked up to the patient in such a manner that they produce readable biofeedback data concerning the patient's brain waves, internal temperatures, blood pressure, pulse, muscle tension, skin resistance, and/or breathing rate. Usually this data is presented in graphic form on a video screen, making it easy to identify and interpret. In some cases, patients can perform this interpretive task on their own and even train themselves to alter their brain and body signals based on the biofeedback they get. Many epileptics have managed to change their brain's electrical activity through biofeedback and, as a result, reduce the number and intensity of their seizures. Migraine headache victims using biofeedback have taught themselves to raise the temperature in their hands, which causes a rerouting of blood to

Color Me Happy

The mind-body connection is forged by perception: What we sense can often influence what we become, even on a physical level. The function of color in interior design offers a simple and direct illustration of this principle.

Warm hues, such as reds, yellows, and oranges, tend to stir the emotions and make an individual more inclined to activity. Restaurateurs, for example, are fond of covering the walls of their establishments with red in order to stimulate appetites. For similar reasons,

yellow is a popular color in household kitchens (where red would usually be too overpowering and dark).

Shades on the cooler side of the spectrum, such as blues, greens, and violets, induce passivity. This makes them highly appropriate for bedrooms or libraries. It also accounts for why light green is so prevalent on the walls of institutions concerned with population control, like schools, hospitals, government offices, and prisons.

the hands that reverses the painful throbbing of blood vessels in their brain.

What medical science is now telling us about the mind-body connection is supplemented by what we're learning from holistic health advocates, who argue that a personally directed, life-style approach to therapy can be just as valuable as a doctor-directed, drugs-surgery-and-machinery approach. Among the specific nonmedical techniques that are proving effective in tapping the mind-body connection are behavior modification, positive thinking, meditation, and visualization. In addition to recouping physical health, these techniques have also been used to develop and improve physical skills, particularly the specialized skills associated with athletic performance.

In this chapter, you'll ex-mance.

In this chapter, you'll examine both scientific and nonscientific insights into the mind-body connection. You'll read about how various stressful events influence your physical well-being and what you can do to counteract that influence. You'll discover ways in which you can increase your body's capabilities through "brain-training." You'll learn some of the truths and fallacies behind such controversial mind-versus-body topics as positive thinking, the placebo effect, and hypochondria. And you'll become more familiar with a new branch of science devoted to studying the mind-body connection—a discipline known professionally as psychoneuroimmunology.

Throughout the human body, a single episode of stress can manifest itself in tangible, often observable ways.

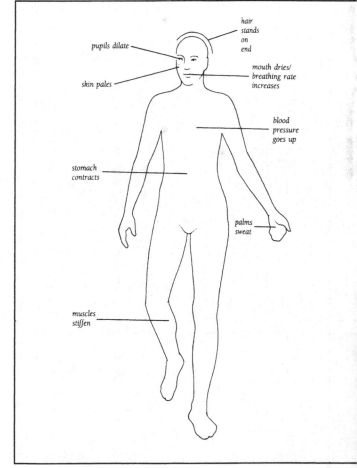

pupils dilate

hair stands on end

mouth dries/ breathing rate increases

skin pales

blood pressure goes up

stomach contracts

palms sweat

muscles stiffen

How Can I Gain More Control Over Stress in My Life?

Although many people find it difficult to believe that the mind can play a major role in causing or curing disease, no one doubts that mental stress can produce physical symptoms. Few of us, however, actually know how stress works, and this ignorance stands in our way of coping with stress effectively.

Science identifies stress as a physiological chain reaction, commonly dubbed the fight-or-flight response, set in motion by the brain whenever it encounters a situation it perceives as demanding, unpleasant, and/or threatening. In a wilder and woollier era of human history, the stress reaction was stirred by the growl of a saber-toothed tiger or the sight of an alien poacher's spear. Today, the same kind of reaction can be provoked by much less physically fearsome events—anything from the squeak of chalk on a blackboard to news of a stock market crash.

Whatever causes the stress, this is what happens in the brain: Upon being faced with an uncomfortable situation, the hypothalamus releases a chemical (commonly abbreviated as CRF) that directs the nearby pituitary gland to secrete adrenocorticotropic hormone (ACTH) that prompts the adrenal glands atop the kidneys to pump corticoid and adrenaline into the bloodstream. Within the brain, corticoid and adrenaline act as neuron stimulants. This full-circle process puts our whole brain and body on red alert.

Because demanding, unpleasant, and/or threatening sit-

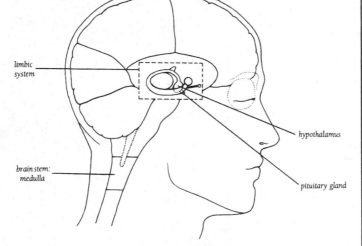

limbic system

brain stem: medulla

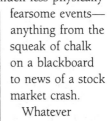

hypothalamus

pituitary gland

uations are inevitable facts of life, so is stress. We're inclined to think of stress as a negative force—an uncomfortable feeling engendered by undesirable events, but it also has a positive dimension. Stress can alert us to dangers we wouldn't otherwise recognize. It can prepare us to function at top capacity when we need to do so. And it can egg us on to solve problems we might otherwise put off, or to exercise our creativity more energetically and productively. Some of us work best under stressful situations, and some of us actively seek high risk, stress-inducing leisure activities—like mountain climbing, hang gliding, or car racing—for the sheer thrill factor.

Stress is undeniably negative, however, if it takes us against our will, if it reaches excessive proportions, or if we deal with it in a clumsy manner. Here are some brainy suggestions for keeping stress in your life under control.

Learn to Recognize and Anticipate Stress Triggers. The more you know about what types of situations can cause you to experience the fight-or-flight response, the more you can work to avoid or manage these situations more adeptly.

First consider major events commonly associated with stress. According to the Life Event Scale published by Dr. T. H. Holmes and Dr. R. H. Rahe in 1976 and based on over 5,000 interviews of people around the world, the ten most stressful crises in a person's life are (in order): death of a spouse or immediate family member, divorce, marital separation, death of a close family member or friend, major personal illness or injury, marriage, being fired or laid off work, major change in the health or behavior of a family member, sexual difficulties, and gaining a new family member.

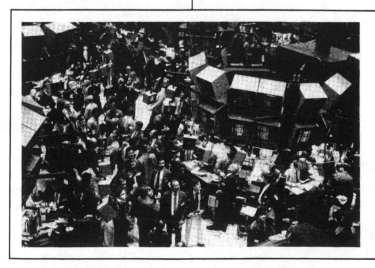

The New York Stock Exchange is a veritable cauldron of stress, which can be productive (technically, "eustress") as well as destructive.

Next, take an inventory of your personal, day-to-day life and consider the things that typically cause you to feel stress. Such things might include worrying about your appearance, having an overcrowded schedule, meeting new people, losing money, dealing with traffic, or handling a particular work responsibility.

Learn to Recognize and Anticipate Physical and Emotional Effects of Stress. It helps to know what to expect when you confront a stressful situation. It also helps to know when you are, in fact, experiencing stress. You may not even realize that stress lies behind certain physical or emotional symptoms unless you make a conscious effort to draw the connection. Common physical symptoms include rapid heartbeat, heavy perspiration, shortening of breath, paling of the skin, tightening of the stomach, tensing of the muscles, clenching of the jaw, and/or more pressure to urinate or defecate. Common emotional symptoms include fear, excitement, restlessness, heightened sensitivity, anger, loneliness, despair, and/or grief.

Work to Minimize or Eliminate Specific Causes of Stress. If you face a major change in your life—the death of a loved one, a marriage, a new job—prepare yourself to go through this transition with as little stress as possible by becoming more informed about it in advance and by planning ahead so that you have plenty of time and resources to help you cope. If a specific person, place, object, or situation regularly inspires stress, take whatever action you can to improve matters: Talk it out with an obnoxious friend or else end the relationship; find some other place to shop that will be cleaner and less hectic; get rid of your outworn yard tools and buy new ones; remodel your kitchen storage space so that it won't be so aggravating to prepare a large meal.

Work to Minimize or Eliminate Specific Effects of Stress. When you're in the tangible grip of the fight-or-flight response, try methodically calming yourself down. Give yourself a break to perform some easygoing activity that you enjoy. As a general treatment for stress, Dr. Herbert Benson of the Mind/Body Clinic at Boston's New England Deaconess Hospital recommends what he calls the relaxation response: Sit comfortably still, close your eyes, and concentrate on a short, soothing word or phrase for ten to twenty minutes. If self-help fails and the effects of stress are bothersomely repetitive or chronic, seek professional advice.

Counterbalance Sources of Stress in Your Life with Sources of Harmony. Develop closer ties to the people you love. Set up dependable routines in your schedule to which you can look forward during times of stress: a few moments each evening in a hot bath, regular nights to eat out, one day per month in bed, seasonal vacations. Create environments around you that are physically and emotionally restorative: a peaceful workspace, a blossom-filled window box you can see from where you eat, a permanent exercise nook. Regularly perform simple tasks that you can be certain will give you a sense of accomplishment.

HYPO-CHONDRIACS

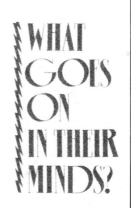

It's a familiar scenario: You read a few facts about a debilitating disease—let's call it "pseudonia." Its symptoms, let's say, are fatigue, dehydration, and/or a light rash. For days to come, every time you feel tired or thirsty, or notice tiny pink bumps on your arm, you get scared. You convince yourself that you *do* feel sick. "What if it's (gasp!) pseudonia?" you wonder.

All of us worry from time to time about falling victim to a particular illness: cancer, heart disease, arthritis, even beriberi. And all of us occasionally have strange physical pains or manifestations that make us think we have a disease, whether we can name it or not. Some people, however, go one giant step further. They may become phobic about one or more specific maladies, taking extreme measures to avoid any possible action or circumstance

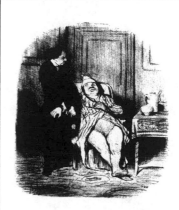

"Oh, Doctor, I'm sure I'm consumptive!" (Honoré Daumier)

that might increase their risk. Or they may agonize over each separate instance of physical discomfort and change, certain that it's a symptom of serious trouble.

We call these one-step-further people hypochondriacs and deride them mercilessly, often telling them that their problems are "all in their head." From a scientific point of view, however, their problems lie in the mind-body connection, and they're painfully real. The chief cause of hypochondria, experts now claim, is an unusually high sensitivity in the brain and nervous system to a wide range of body sensations. Dr. Arthur Barsky of Harvard Medical School recently studied 115 patients who came to a Boston clinic complaining of respiratory infections. He discovered that those patients who described symptoms far worse than indicated by medical examination were also atypically sensitive to physical stimulation in general. Their physiological responses to noise, heat, cold, and hunger were much stronger than normal, and their verbal accounts of past body-related experiences were much more vivid and detailed.

Yet another potential source of hypochondria is social conditioning. It can begin with the nuclear family: If parents are unduly solicitous whenever their child is sick, then the child may grow up to be overly concerned about the threat of illness. Even more insidious is the potential influence of the culture as a whole. According to Dr. Susan Baur of the University of California, there's a mild hypochondria prevalent throughout American society— "irrational health worries that affect so many people that not to be preoccupied seems bizarre." She cites "weight-watcher's hypochondria" and "fitness hypochondria" in particular. Many people become so obsessed about avoiding calories in their diet and adding miles to their jogs that they wind up endangering their health instead of enhancing it.

Ironically, Barksy contends, hypochondria may be increasing as a direct result of improvements in health care. "Having come to imagine that somewhere there is a treatment for almost everything that ails us," he notes, "we experience refractory symptoms as a mistake, an injustice, a failure of medical care." For the true hypochondriac, this translates into endless rounds from one specialist to another, and, logically enough, as the perceived symptom

Pain, Pain, Go Away

"Where does it hurt?" the dentist asked Bertrand Russell, the famous English philosopher and mathematician. "In my mind, of course," Russell replied. True, the danger signal we know as pain is set in motion by neurochemicals at the site of an injury, disease, or illness, but the pain sensation itself is a highly subjective experience—dependent to a great degree on how the brain and the mind perceive it.

Sometimes one's expectations make all the difference in whether a pain is intense or not. Familiar kinds of "pain" signals are seldom as scary and bothersome as ones we've never encountered before. Signals that can be explained are not as alarming as signals that lack an explanation.

At other times one's perception of pain is heavily influenced by surrounding circumstances. If we're absorbed in a mentally and/or physically demanding project at the time the signal strikes, we're far less likely to notice it and develop an intolerant sensitivity to it than we are if we've got nothing else to think about. If loud music, a cold wind, or a crowd of friends is competing with the signal for our brain's attention, then any pain we register can be significantly diminished.

receives more and more scrutiny, it grows more and more intense.

A final factor possibly contributing to hypochondria—one that gets more than its fair share of credit—is psychological maladjustment. Some therapists tell us that hypochondria can be a desperate strategy for attracting sympathy; others explain it as a willful desire to attribute bodily aches and pains to disease, rather than aging, neglect, overexertion, or emotional stress. Whatever the specific issue, therapists are anxious to avoid the counterproductive stigma associated with the term "hypochondriac," and so they officially call the victim a "somatizer" (soma is Greek for "body").

If the source of the hypochondriac's problem does seem to be psychological in nature, then extensive psychological therapy is the answer. Otherwise, a more common-sense mental coaching can work wonders. The first step to a cure is for the victim to recognize that he or she does have a built-in tendency to overreact. The second step is to get the victim to accept that he or she will have to live in some degree of discomfort that can't be helped. We all have to do this, in fact, but for a hypochondriac, that discomfort can be much stronger and therefore more difficult to tolerate. The third and final step is for the victim to learn as much as he or she can about the way in which the physical body works, concentrating specifically on diseases that he or she fears and on the mind-body connection in general. Hypochondria is bad enough without being compounded by suspicion and ignorance. The truth in this situation can definitely go a long way to setting the victim free.

Keeping these factors in mind, here are some tips for pain control.

Establish the Reason Behind the Pain. Consider not only the physical source but also any psychological or situational forces that may be augmenting the pain. For particularly baffling pains, professional counsel can be reassuring and pain-reducing in its own right.

Disassociate Yourself from the Pain Signal. Many people practice visualizing their pain as contained within a box in one part of their body. This helps them to avoid the panic-ridden "I feel bad all over" response. Others imagine they are looking at themselves and their pain from an outside perspective—beside their real body or ten feet above it. People in isolated areas who must perform quasi-surgical procedures on one of their own body parts (such as sewing a gash in the leg) typically think of that body part as an inanimate object.

Seek Distraction from Your Pain. Try to occupy your mind with something else so that you are not so conscious of the pain signal. Paint a wall or a picture. Watch a funny movie. Take a stroll through the park. Chat with a friend.

How Can I Use My Brain to Enhance My Physical Prowess?

During the last two minutes before their first run in the 1988 Winter Olympics, members of the U.S. bobsled team stood silently by the side of their sled with their eyes closed. They weren't praying. They were visualizing every detail of the run as if they were already making it. On or off camera, this kind of disciplined mental rehearsal has become a regular and rewarding exercise for many successful Olympians. During the 1988 Summer

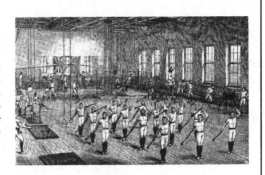
Olympics, the American diver Greg Louganis, a gold-medal winner for springboard and platform diving, "mind-scripted" each dive an estimated forty times, sometimes imagining it in real time, sometimes going through it in slow motion, to check out how different parts of his body behaved and felt at different moments.

Brain-training, as it's now being called, acknowledges the role that *all* brain functions play in the physical performance of the body. The neurochemical stimulation of muscles, organs, and glands may be the brain's basic and most obvious contribution to body movement, but today's sports psychologists tell us that if we want to execute a specific activity as effectively as possible, we need to gain more control over the way the brain processes factors of consciousness, memory, intelligence, and emotions that relate to that activity. Mentally living through a specific physical challenge in advance allows our brain to prepare itself for optimum functioning at all levels when the time comes to perform that challenge for real.

What's good for athletic endeavors is also good for any other type of physical endeavor. Chefs-in-training at the Culinary Institute of America in Hyde Park, New York, are routinely directed by some of their instructors to rehearse a new recipe or cooking technique in their minds, step by step, before trying it out in the kitchen. Prior to using an unfamiliar or difficult surgical procedure on a patient, the nationally known urologist Dr. Ira Sharlip sits quietly in his study and mentally enacts each step. If he has any trouble with a particular movement, he consults colleagues, books, and videotapes until he can imagine doing it easily and completely. Louganis himself, now a post-Olympian, is applying brain-training to his fledgling career as a singer, dancer, and actor.

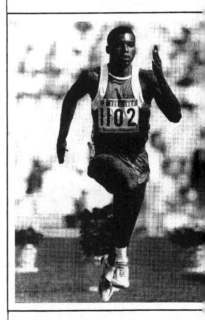

Track-and-field superstar Carl Lewis works with the equivalent of video games to develop the mental concentration powers he applies to the Olympic Games.

One of the most vociferous exponents of brain-training is Dr. Richard M. Suinn of Colorado State University, who has demonstrated that imagining an event can elicit virtually any type of neural response. In an experiment conducted early in the 1980s, Suinn electronically monitored the muscle activity of an Alpine ski racer as the racer sat in a chair narrating his own visualization of a race on a specific course. "I found that I could match his verbal description with bursts of muscle activity recorded during the visualization," Suinn recalls. "For example, he described an area where he jumped into the air, and we got a burst of activity at that point. When he described a bumpy part of the course, there was activity again."

Not all brain-training consists of imagining a physical activity in realistic detail. Dr. Shane Murphy of the United States Olympic Training Center at Colorado Springs believes that the most important element of brain-training is to visualize the activity in the context of success. Some athletes, like the U.S. track-and-field superstar Carl Lewis, keep their minds focused on what they want as a *result* of their physical performance. "I picture myself at the other end of the jump—having soared through the air and made a good landing," Lewis says. "I don't ever remember the seconds that I'm actually in the air."

Other brain-trainers opt for a poetic, "psych-up" approach. A skater for the Ice Capades, for example, always envisions swallowing a star and having its energy burst inside her when she makes her entrance. As a jogger travels his route, he visualizes a rubber band of light pulling him from the beginning to the end. A weight lifter pretends during a workout that he is simultaneously making and watching a perfect training film to replace the last one he "made."

Suinn claims that visualization constitutes a new form of learning, along with classical conditioning, in which we learn by experience; operant conditioning, in which we learn by performing instructional exercises; and vicarious conditioning, in which we learn by observing others. Whatever visualization represents, it has made a noteworthy leap from the ethereal realm of mystical contemplation to the sweaty world of muscle and bone.

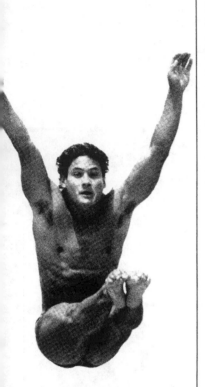

Greg Louganis, twenty-eight years old during the 1988 Summer Olympics in Seoul, has been using visualization to increase his athletic prowess since he was a sixteen-year-old competing at the 1976 Summer Olympics in Montreal (where he captured a silver medal in diving).

THE PLACEBO EFFECT

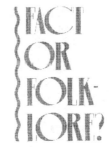
FACT OR FOLK-LORE?

In the late 1950s, a man with life-threatening cancer begged his doctor to give him the experimental drug Krebiozen, then being widely heralded as a "miracle cure." It took just one dose, and his advanced tumors went into swift and complete remission. Later, the man read reports suggesting that Krebiozen was not a bona fide cancer treatment, and almost immediately his tumors reappeared. Knowing that nothing else could be done, his doctor gave the man what he said was an improved Krebiozen. In truth, it was only water, but, wonder of wonders, the tumors started shrinking again. The man's health continued to improve until he learned that Krebiozen had been declared worthless once and for all by the U.S. Food and Drug Administration. Within days, the man died.

What we see in this well-documented and highly publicized case is an extraordinary example of the placebo effect. We tend to think of a placebo (from the Latin, "I shall please") as a "sugar pill," something harmless that will satisfy a sick person's demand for medicine when nothing legitimate is available, or that can be used in a drug experiment to create a blind control group. Actually, medical science is now in the process of proving what shamans, homeopaths, and worried mothers have always known to be true—that an individual's beliefs and expectations can set off an internal healing response that has the power to be as effective as any other form of therapy, if not more effective.

How, specifically, does the placebo effect work? So far, details are few. In a number of experiments, the placebo effect has been associated with an increase in the brain's production of endorphins. If an endorphin-neutralizing drug like naloxone is administered after a placebo, any loss of pain the subject has experienced is reversed. Placebos can also cause a decrease in any or all of the brain's anxiety signals to the body. The combined result of endorphin stimulation and

In cultures throughout the world, the shaman was—and, in places like the Amazon region, equitorial Africa, and Borneo, still is—a healer who relies heavily on the power of faith to effect physical cures.

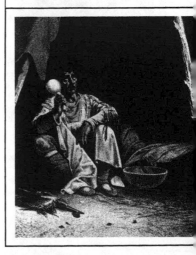

anxiety suppression would certainly enhance a sick person's sense of well-being and might even physiologically enable natural recovery mechanisms to function better. But that still leaves big questions regarding why the placebo effect works in some situations and not others, and how it occasionally causes such dramatic reversals of terminal illnesses as the one described above.

Dr. Jon Levine of the University of California at San Francisco believes that the context in which the placebo is administered contributes significantly to the placebo's success. "The wearing of a white coat by the doctor, along with a stethoscope and other medical accoutrements," he claims, "will help provide an image to the patient which suggests that the interactions should produce a therapeutic effect." This tendency to conform to the expectations of authorities is called the Pygmalion effect. Similarly, the spiritual climate and reputation surrounding the famous Shrine of Lourdes in France may have made the difference in triggering many of the spontaneous, scientifically inexplicable cures that have been validated there by the resident International Medical Committee.

We may not be able to make placebos function precisely when and how we want them to function, but the mere fact that the placebo effect does have the potential of working is one more piece of evidence that our mindset influences those brain and body mechanisms that determine our health. Realizing this, we all need to look at our illness-related beliefs and expectations much more closely, nurturing the ones that we feel offer the most promise and amending the ones that appear to stand in the way of our recovery.

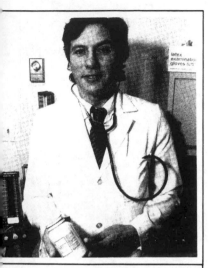

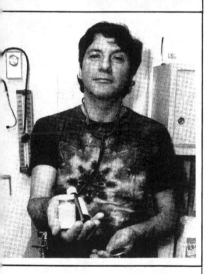

Which doctor is more likely to make *you* feel better, even if their prescriptions are identical?

Can Positive Thinking Help Me Live a Longer, Healthier Life?

The notion that a healthy mind means a healthy body strikes many people as a recent invention. The phrase "positive thinking" itself, suggesting the deliberate cultivation of a happy frame of mind, was coined only forty years ago by Dr. Norman Vincent Peale of New York City's Marble Collegiate Church, who went on to write a

McCarthyism: A Social Malady

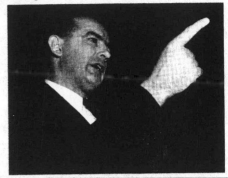

A classic "Type A, hostile" personality, Joseph McCarthy, a Republican U.S. Senator from Wisconsin, gained worldwide attention in the early 1950s by stirring up hatred against Communists and thereby ruining the careers of many law-abiding Americans. Television broadcasts of his Congressional hearings investigating alleged Communist infiltration of the U.S. Army exposed the near-pathological nature of his hostility and brought about his public disgrace in 1954. He died in 1957 at the age of forty-nine, a victim of liver failure attributed to heavy drinking.

string of popular books on the subject. And New Age philosophy asserts its newness by preaching the two-way interdependence of attitude and illness, most successfully and controversially in the 1986 bestseller *Love, Medicine, and Miracles* by Yale surgeon Dr. Bernie Siegel.

Modern sounding it may be, but the idea goes back at least 3,000 years, when Vedic literature first defined our physical being as a projection of our inner consciousness. And now scientists, after amassing several centuries of empirical evidence, are coming up with solid research in support of that ancient definition.

In a 1989 address to the American Heart Association, Dr. Redford Williams of Duke University revealed the results of a twenty-five-year study indicating that hostile people are likely to have shorter lives than people who are good-natured. His study followed the medical histories of 118 lawyers who had taken the Minnesota Multiphasic Personality Inventory (MMPI), a well regarded and widely used diagnostic instrument, during law school. Those subjects who had scored high on hostility proved to be five times as likely to die before fifty as their classmates who had scored low on hostility.

Williams's research has shed new light on the groundbreaking Type A versus Type B theory proposed in the 1970s by two San Francisco cardiologists, Meyer Friedman and Ray Rosenman. Based on their patients' files, Friedman and Rosenman concluded that people who are generally intense, aggressive, and ambitious (Type A personalities) are much more likely to experience strokes and

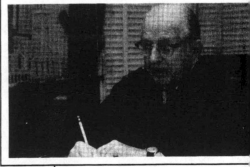

Dr. Norman Vincent Peale's "positive thinking" books have been translated into fifty-three languages and have influenced more grass-roots experimentation with attitude reform than any other body of work produced in the years since World War II.

heart attacks than people who are generally easygoing, co-operative, and modest (Type B personalities). While conceding his indebtedness to this theory, Williams is convinced that it goes a bit too far. "We can now state with some confidence," he says, "that of all the aspects originally described as making up the global Type A pattern, only those related to hostility are really prone to heart disease."

As interpreted by psychologists, hostility includes the following attitudes and behaviors: anger, leading to antagonistic deeds, gestures, or words (for example, "What do you think you're doing?" or "Look at that crazy driver!"); suspicion, expressed in such activities as covertly watching to make sure people do what you want them to do; and cynicism, which can take the form of always assuming the worst about a person or a situation. Hostility is not necessarily a part of being a workaholic or being competitive, nor can the latter traits be directly associated with any higher risk of disease or early death.

A contemporaneous and altogether different body of research suggests that unemotional people are more prone to contract cancer, while emotional people are more prone to suffer heart disease. Summarizing the results of three long-term studies—one in Yugoslavia (1,353 subjects) and two in West Germany (872 and 1,942 subjects), the distinguished European psychologist Dr. Ronald Grossarth-Matichek established four different types of personalities:

- *Type 1 (underaroused)*—people who are relatively passive and succumb easily to depression
- *Type 2 (overaroused)*—people who are relatively demonstrative and typically respond to difficulties with anger or frustration
- *Type 3 (ambivalent)*—people who alternate between Type 1 and Type 2 behaviors
- *Type 4 (autonomous)*—people who are emotionally well adjusted and not overly dependent on other people or outside situations for their self-esteem and happiness.

Consistently, the people who fell in the Type 1 category were far more likely to die of cancer than heart disease. In a third of the study groups, the ratio was as high as five to one. By contrast, Type 2 people inevitably proved far more likely to die of heart disease than cancer. Again, in a third of the study groups, the ratio was about five to one. Neither Type 3 nor Type 4 subjects revealed any pronounced tendency toward cancer as opposed to heart disease.

Taken together, the Williams studies and the Grossarth-Matichek studies support the idea that maintaining a positive, nonhostile, and emotionally balanced mind-set can, indeed, help you to live a longer, healthier life. Here are some mind-mellowing tips.

- Monitor how you're thinking and behaving, and try to stop negative thoughts and behaviors in their tracks. Ask yourself: Why am I thinking or behaving this way? What's the positive alternative? What might make it easier for me—now and in the future—to think or act positively in this type of situation?
- Seek diversion when you get depressed or frustrated about a certain person or situation. Involve yourself with another person or situation that will take your mind off your troubles.
- As a general rule, practice forgiving whenever possible, listening more patiently to what others have to say, laughing at yourself when you behave inappropriately, and expressing your point of view calmly during disagreements.
- Treat your brain well. Make sure that you always get sufficient sleep each night, that you build several periods of relaxation into each day, and that you avoid overindulgence in neurochemically toxic substances like nicotine, caffeine, alcohol, and refined sugar. This will help your brain function as its physiological, intellectual, and emotional best.

◆◆◆◆◆◆◆◆◆◆

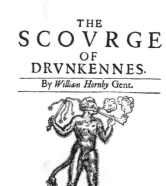

THE
SCOVRGE
OF
DRVNKENNES.
By *William Hornby* Gent.

LONDON,
Printed by G. E ı ᴅ, for *Thomas Bayſie*, and are to be folde
at his Shop, in the Middle-Row in Holborne,
neere vnto *Staple-Inne,* ı 6 ı 8.

Published in London in 1618, this pamphlet entitled "The Scourge of Drunkennes [i.e., Drunkenness]" actually refers to tobacco-smoking—a habit freshly imported from native America that was already being recognized as having sour effects on the brain.

PSYCHO-
NEURO-
IMMUNO-
LOGY

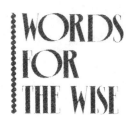

It helps to divide this tongue twister into its parts: psycho—the mind; neuro—nerve cells or the nervous system; and immuno—the immune system, that complex network of cells, glands, and organs that attacks disease-causing microbes. In 1975, Dr. Robert Ader of the University of Rochester coined the term "psychoneuroimmunology" to identify a fascinating new scientific discipline—the study of how one's beliefs and emotions influence one's brain chemistry and one's state of health.

Ader, a psychologist, and his colleague Dr. Nicholas Cohen, an immunologist, laid the foundation for this discipline in a series of experiments with rats. First, they gave the rats saccharine water, and then they injected them with a drug causing temporary illness. Eventually, all they had to do was to give the rats saccharine water and they got sick. Their minds were telling their immune systems how to behave based on what they'd been conditioned to believe. Later, Dr. Herbert Spector of the National Institutes of Health proved that such conditioning works both ways. He repeatedly exposed mice to the smell of camphor followed by an immune-boosting drug. Eventually, just the smell of camphor alone would demonstrably increase their immune systems. Sometimes, it only took nine repetitions for the effect to take hold.

Since these startling experiments, many scientists have concluded that the mind, the brain, and the immune system are physiologically linked in a back-and-forth communication system far more intricate than orthodox Western medicine has ever imagined. Experts have known for quite a while that both the brain and the immune system communicate through chemical signals and can remember facts (the immune system's memory enables vaccinations to work). They've also long been aware that the brain's hypothalamus serves not only as a transmitter of emotional signals, but also as a regulator of the immune system. But now the boldest psychoneuroimmunologists claim that the immune system's white blood cells are, in fact, almost identical in structure and capabilities to neurons.

Research conducted by Dr. Candace Pert at the National Institute of Mental Health has established that white cells, like brain cells, can send or receive a wide variety of messages and can make or discharge a number of hormones. The implications of her work are astounding. In effect, Pert says, white blood cells may be "bits of the brain floating around the body," with the ability to generate emotions and respond to them just like neurons and with constant "walkie-talkie" brain contact. Further research by Pert has shown that two of the main body organs utilized by the immune system—the thymus and the spleen—are connected by an extraordinarily dense network of nerve cells to the brain. Presumably, this strong connective bridge would make comunication between the nervous system and the immune system all the more intimate.

Psychoneuroimmunology remains a highly nebulous and controversial discipline at the moment, but it holds a great deal of promise. *If* science is able to discover further ways in which the mind, the brain, and the immune system dialogue with each other, and *if* science can devise methods for controlling this dialogue, then the world of medicine will undergo revolutionary change. Psychoneuroimmunologists are especially excited about the new possibilities for drug therapy, for disease prevention, and for the treatment of psychosensitive disorders like allergies and lupus.

At present, Pert is specifically interested in finding a psychoneuroimmunological cure for AIDS, which she believes is a disease rooted in the disruption of communication between the mind, the brain, and the immune system. To facilitate this search, she and her husband/colleague Dr. Michael Ruff recently founded their own biotechnology company called Peptide Design. As more and more scientific pioneers commit themselves to this challenging field, psychoneuroimmunology (now occasionally abbreviated as PNI) may soon become a household word.

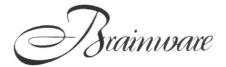

Brainware

Electromyograph

One of medical science's most exciting biofeedback machines, the electromyograph (EMG) has performed wonders in helping patients achieve better control over healthy muscles and, in some cases, regain the use of diseased ones. Electrical sensors are placed on the skin directly over a muscle. The electrical activity produced by the cells of that muscle when they are activated can then be detected, amplified, and displayed on an oscilloscope, which is a monitor much like a television screen. By executing various maneuvers to try to affect this electrical activity, patients "teach" their brains to use alternate neural passages to move the muscle. The process almost always proves therapeutic for simple spasms and strains, and it can frequently be valuable in treating such complicated neuromuscular disorders as palsy and stroke-induced paralysis.

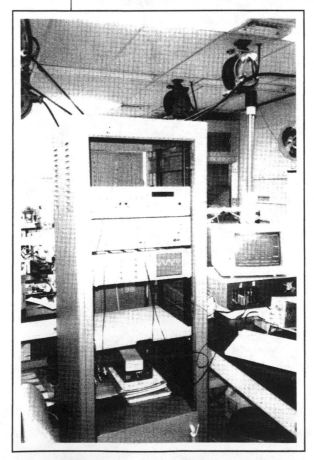

Bridges to Greater Professional Success

Concerned about minimizing interpersonal stress among crew members on long space missions, NASA hired psychologist Taibi Kahler to develop a diagnostic instrument that could identify potential stress triggers according to different personality types. The result was a computer software program that is now being marketed to the general public under the title Bridges to Greater Professional Success. First, the user answers a series of questions to establish his or her particular personality type (or the personality type of someone else) among six models: reactor, workaholic, persister, dreamer, promoter, or rebel. Then the program continues in an interactive mode to offer more information about (a) what kinds of stressful experiences that personality type may have, and how to manage those experiences; (b) what types of stressful experiences may occur in interactions with other personality types, and how to manage those experiences. According to its devotees, the program functions as an ongoing "brain trust" capable of responding meaningfully to any tricky situation, general or specific.

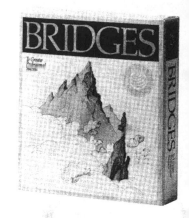

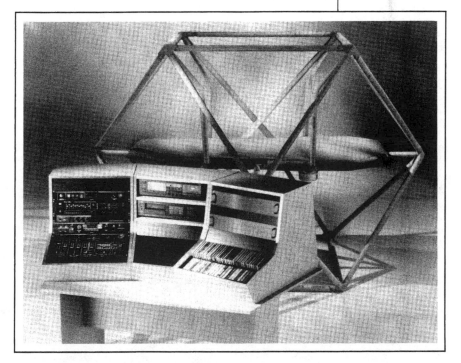

Genesis System

The Genesis System is a brain-gym biofeedback machine with a difference: You can use it not only as a relaxation device but also as an exercise device. A bed is mounted horizontally within a hexagonal framework that has two exercise crossbars. Triphonic speakers play the music of your choice, and acoustical sensors read which frequencies in the music have the most beneficial impact on the electrical activity in your brain. Vibrating transducers within the bed transmit only those "good vibrations." The combination of the speaker music and the selectively transmitted vibration frequencies gives the user's mind and body a "surround-sound" massage. Clients choosing soft, mellow music for relaxation describe the experience as "floating like musical notes." Clients choosing up-tempo music for exercise (for example, disco songs or the Rocky theme) report being able to do pull-ups, push-ups, and sit-ups with much more stamina and precision than usual.

PHOTO CREDITS

Mind Mirror, Coherent Communications, Inc.
p. 65

Robyn Feller
pp. 73, 125

Adapted from drawing, National Institute of Neurological
Disorders and Stroke, National Institute of Health, Bethesda, MD
p. 82

The Museum of Modern Art/Film Stills Archive
pp. 85, 89, 131

Subsidiary of Psion PLC
p. 96

Chronos Software, Inc.
p. 97

R + R Associates, Inc.
p. 97

Office of Scientific and Health Reports
p. 100

UPI/Bettmann Newsphotos
pp. 109, 114, 157, 164, 167

Hi-Tech Innovation Corporation, Dr. Yoshiro NakaMats
p. 124

Electromedical Products, Inc.
p. 125

Photo Researchers, Inc.
© Will McIntyre, p. 135
© Susan Rosenberg, p. 142

Hammacher Schlemmer
p. 148

Tranquil Times, Inc.
p. 149

Jim Gautier
p. 152

Bio-Feedback Systems, Inc.
p. 153

Reuters/Bettmann Newsphotos
p. 163

Seth Eastman
p. 165

Mount Sinai Medical School
photo by Robyn Feller, p. 172

Three-Sixty Pacific, Inc.
p. 173

Profit Technology, Inc.
p. 173

INDEX

Stress (*cont.*)
  emotional symptoms, 158
  headaches resulting from, 23
  minimizing, 158
  nature of, 156
  physical symptoms, 158
  productive, 157
  relief, 4
  and schizophrenia, 29
  software for analysis, 173
  treatment, 158–59
Stroke victims, memore improvement, 81
Stuttering, hemisphere interaction, 10
Subliminal messages
  effectiveness, 61–62
  in visual formats, 62–63
Substance abuse, chemical basis, 18
Suinn, Richard M., 164
Superego, 44–45
Superspace, 64
Synapse, 6–7
Synchro-Energizer, 4, 65
Synchronicity, 46

Taste, linked to memory, 71
Temporal lobe, 5, 7
Tension headaches, 23–24
Terman, Michael, 146
Thalamus, 128
THC, effect on brain, 21
Therapy
  behaviroal approach, 133
  cognitive approach, 133
  holistic approach, 155

interpersonal approach, 133
Theta waves, 7
Thiamine, effect on brain, 77
Thought
  PET scan showing, 100
  physiological changes resulting, 100
Time-gap experiences, 34
Toxic headaches, 24–25
Tranquilite machine, 149
Transcranial electrotherapy, 125
Tryptophan, effect on brain, 41
Twilight Learning System, Model TL-1, 153
Tyrosine, 41

Unconscious mind
  defined, 44–45
  personal versus collective, 45

Vascular headaches, categories, 23–25
Vinpocetine, 81
Vision, brain area controlling, 7
Visualization, 144, 155
  See also Brain-training
Vitamins, importance to intelligence, 116
Voodoo, 152

Wehr, Thomas, 146
Weil, Andrew, 35
Wenger, Win, 11
Williams, Redford, 167
Wurtman, Judith, 40–41
Wurtman, Richard, 40–41